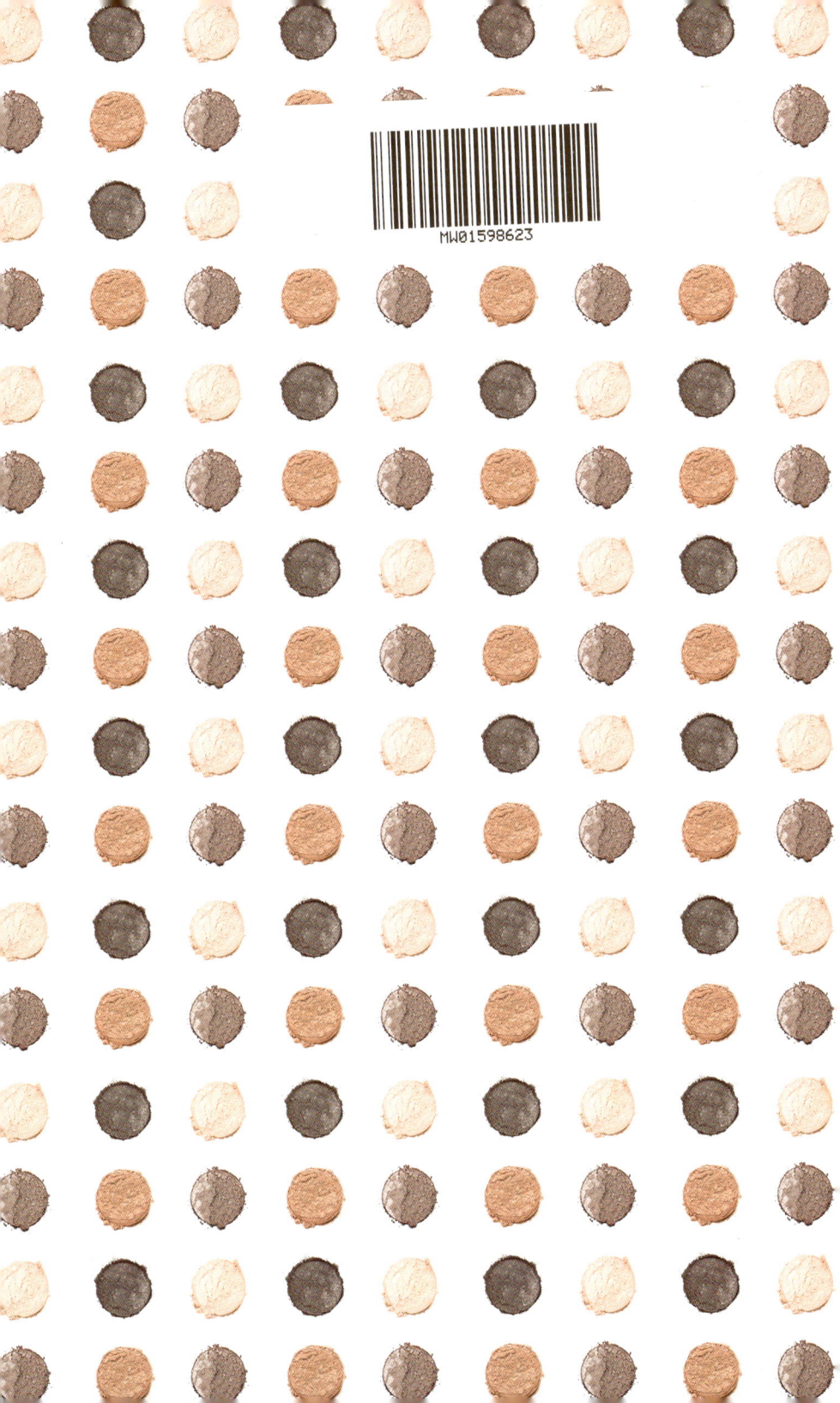

MW01598623

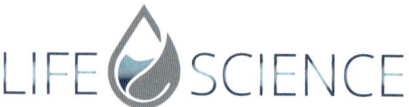

Copyright © 2018
Life Science Publishing
1.800.336.6308
www.DiscoverLSP.com

Printed in the United States of America
10 9 8 7 6 5 4 3 2 1

Foreword

We all want the best that nature can provide. That's why I'm so pleased with the Savvy Minerals® product line from Young Living. It is a wonderful new way to use essential-oil infused products and clean, Seed to Seal™ solutions that protect us in such crucial ways. Besides what we put in our bodies, nothing concerns most of us as much as what we put on our faces.

At the age of 21, I was told that I would not live to see 30 because of a serious autoimmune disease. My only chance at survival? Over 15 months of grueling, heartbreaking chemotherapy. It was a long-hard battle and at one point, the treatments caused my skin to bleed and ooze. This happened all over my body, but more alarmingly, it happened on my face, heartbreakingly leaving facial scars that I've dealt with for the remainder of my adult life.

Beauty, skin care, and cosmetics have been my quest ever since this experience. I have felt insecurity, personal doubt, and have struggled with coming to terms with the traumatic experience—all during that pivotal time in my life when I ought to have felt I was at my most young and beautiful.

To top it off, the condition left me highly sensitive and even allergic to many simple things. (I can't even use aloe!) Though I've tried everything possible (and I'm relentlessly optimistic), I rarely find a skin product that works for me (the way it's intended) or doesn't cause me to have a reaction or breakout.

The blessing of Young Living's essential oils has really changed that for me. My skin is in better shape, having used these marvelous tools, than it has ever been since my early twenties. Through the combination of oils, ART® skin care, and now Savvy Minerals, I can truly leave the self-consciousness and trepidation behind.

When Young Living launched this line in 2017, I raised my hands and cheered! Now we all can feel a little safer, a little more secure, and a little more hopeful that the face we show the world is one that's toxin-free. I hope you find Jill's tips and information useful as you explore the Savvy line and share it with the people in your life.

I would love to say we've met, but if all you know of me is the picture in this book, I hope to meet you soon! I've been told that my energy and passion are contagious. If that's the case, I hope you catch them both...

Love. Learn. Share.

XO XO

Troie Battles

Troie Storms-Battles

Author Message

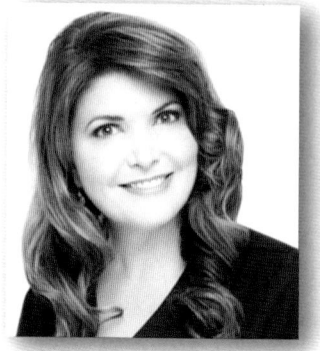

I can remember the first time I put on my mother's lipstick as a child. It had that strange waxy smell that only a petroleum-based product of the early 70s could have. (Any of you who are of a certain age will know exactly what I'm talking about. You can still smell and experience such wonders at a dollar store or the bottom-shelf of your local drugstore!)

Things have come a long way since then. We now know what products look natural on skin, which ones have strange chemicals, and which ones are better left alone. We've gone from being as unnatural as possible for the purpose of achieving that outré—yet trendy—look to being concerned not only about what we put *in* our bodies, but also what we put *on* them.

My experience with Young Living is much like most people. I received a present in the form of a really wonderful essential oil, tried a diffuser, and the rest is history!

My lifelong journey with beauty is a much longer story, full of it's own twists and turns. I was always drawn to hair and makeup from a young age, and even graduated from high school early to attend cosmetology school and begin what's been a 30+-year career in the beauty field.

This immediately brought me to the great adventure of entrepreneurship and sharing beauty. I got married young, had two wonderful children, and then opened a full salon in my home so that I could be near to my kids.

As my kids grew up and time went on, I started to be a little concerned about aging. *Who doesn't fall into that trap?* I wanted to do something that spoke to women my age and decided to go back to school and become an esthetician. After all, I was already accustomed to helping people take care of their skin, hair, and makeup. What was one more step?

It was—and still is—a growing industry with a lot of opportunity. I thought, becoming a Master Esthetician will open a lot of doors—and it did! I was fortunate enough to sign with the largest medical spa group in the Intermountain West.

Being a part of that industry opened my eyes to amazing modern advances. It also opened my eyes to a lot of pain and to a lot of high expecations from people looking to rediscover their youth. They either wanted to turn back the clock or stop it altogether. In working with clients, I experimented with different brands of skin care, makeup, and recovery programs. This was especially a concern since so many of them were having relatively invasive procedures.

I began to see a toll that this takes on the skin, the body, the psyche, and the human soul. Most of us intuitively know that staying closer to Mother Nature just feels more balanced. As a result, if and when I have been able to *opt* for a more natural product,

I do. Any time I can *recommend* something that's environmentally sound and clean, I absolutely will!

That's what is so exciting about Young Living's Savvy Minerals. This is a product that carries Young Living's Seed to Seal™ guarantee! It's chance for all of us to take that more natural approach, that step toward beauty that finally turns away from the Ancient Roman and Egyptian practice of putting lead on the face. It's a chance to marry true health with true beauty.

Some might call beauty *vanity*, but I just see it as a creative way of giving people a more equal playing field. We may not be able to choose our looks when we are born, but we certainly can look at the beauty in ourselves and put our best foot forward. As the famous makeup artist Wayne Goss says, *"No amount of makeup can cover up an ugly soul."*

My own daughter recently graduated from college, got married, and is now ready to have a child of her own. I want them to have all the knowledge that I didn't in my beauty career. We're living in an age of women finding their voice and defining their empowerment . It's about time we embrace the moment and make choices about our health and beauty that don't sacrifice our longevity and quality of life.

I love the Savvy Minerals concept of *Buildable*, *Blendable*, and *Forgiving*. If only the world were more that way, we'd probably be a lot better off! Let's use that mantra to make it more beautiful together!

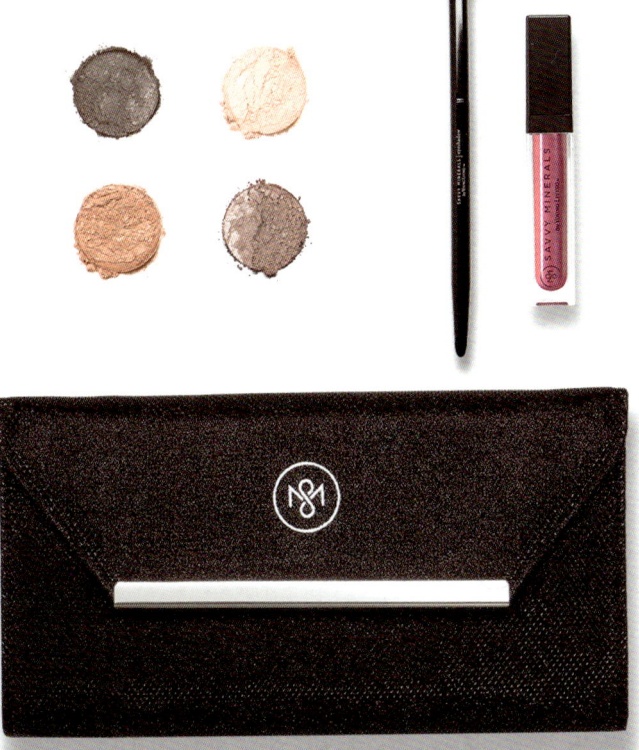

Note About Purity

It is unfortunate that profit has taken priority over health. All too often, essential oils in the marketplace are diluted with solvents or chemicals. These synthetics and hybrids are not pure, nor are they natural. The essential oils we advocate in the Aroma series are only of the utmost, certified quality. We never advocate a product that may damage health or interfere with healing.

That said, essential oils have been used for thousands of years and have helped countless people to live healthier lives. As publishers of the most sought-after text about essential oils, the Essential Oil Desk Reference, we want to make as much information as easily accessible to you and the people you love.

It is with this spirit of education and sharing that we have compiled and summarized many of the specialized volumes we publish. Always take the time to read, study, and share the things you learn. Use good judgment as you add essential oils into your healthy lifestyle.

As Mary Young has said:

"Often times, we think we are helping someone by telling them what to do or giving them direction or advice about a problem that person may have. However, we take on a huge responsibility to give advice when we are not the expert or don't have the license that allows us to give advice. Besides that, if we give advice and then that advice doesn't work, that person may become angry with us and can accuse us of misdiagnosing, misunderstanding, and wasting their time and money.

In the world of essential oils, much information is available. If you are going to use any natural product, I suggest that you research all avenues possible and learn as much as you can for yourself, and then you be the one to decide how you will use any particular product.

It doesn't matter what you are going to eat, put on your skin, breathe, or even soak in, learning as much about your product is the most intelligent and safest thing you can do for yourself. The more information you have, the better choices you will make. After you study and research it for yourself, you may decide you don't want the very thing you thought you were excited about; but that is your decision, not someone else's decision about what you should do.

If you find something that interests you and you are uncertain, ask your doctor or someone educated in the field of health and nutrition. Ask their opinion to add to your knowledge bank. Look on the Internet to learn what research institutes, wellness centers, government agencies, the Surgeon General, and even the FDA have to say. You don't have to agree, but it is to your advantage to know what they say.

It is your responsibility to be responsible for yourself. It is your God-given right to search, read, study, and decide how you will feed and take care of your own body. Be independent and be wise."

--- From A Thought From Mary,
    Mary Young 2016

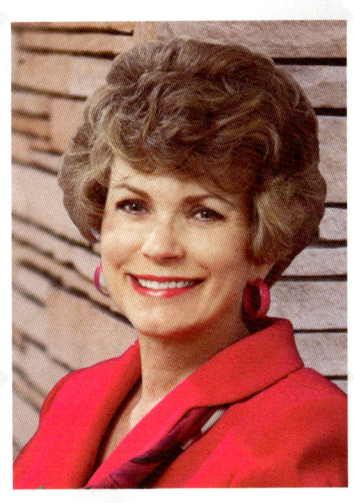

Table Of Contents

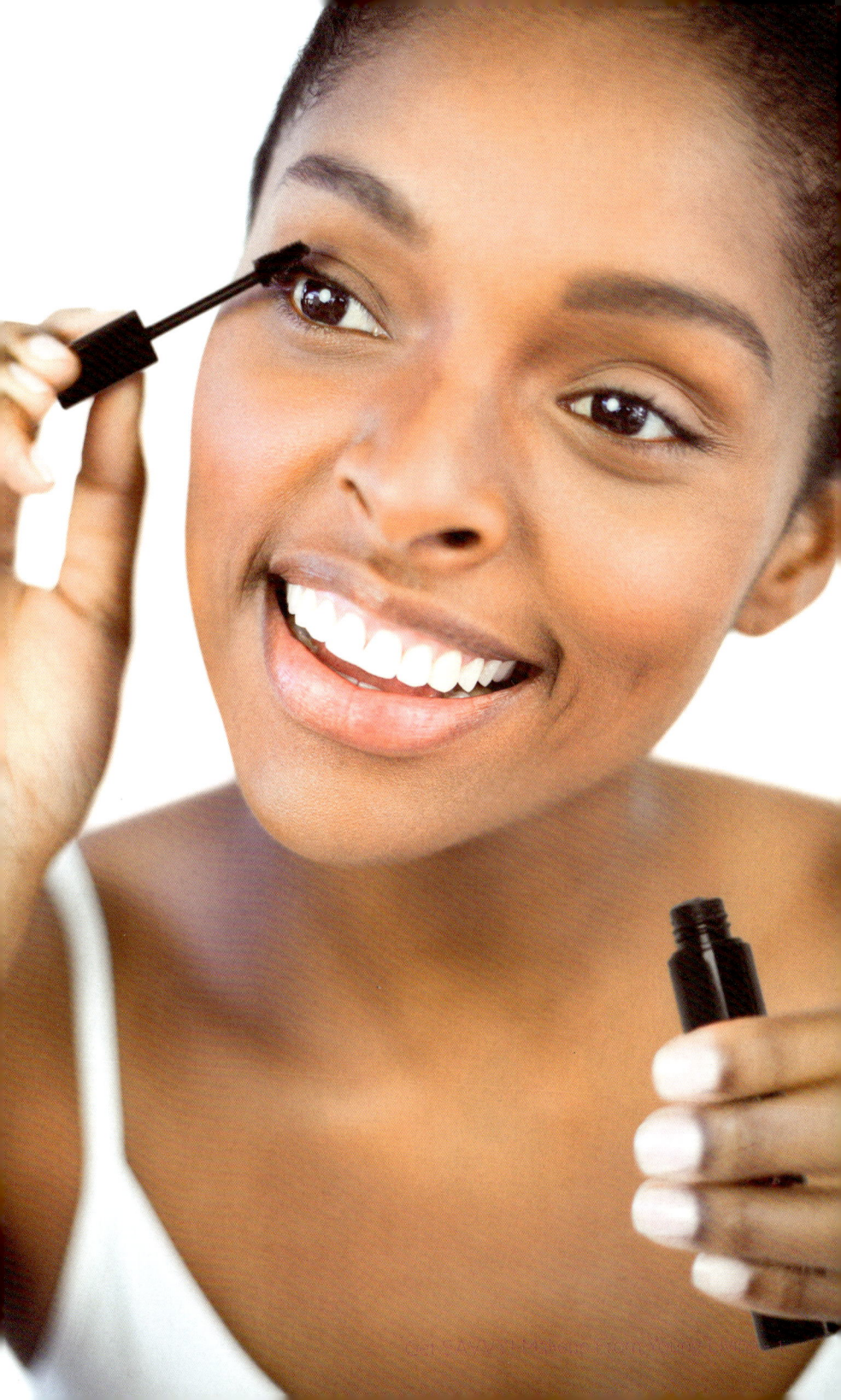

Why Makeup?

There are many people who weren't really brought up wearing makeup. Either their mothers didn't wear it, or they just felt it was artificial and didn't really value the trend or "the look." It didn't really speak to them. What's more, they wanted to be valued for their achievements or their contributions, not for how they looked.

Much of what's portrayed in magazines or glamour shoots isn't real life. In fact, most of it the average person wouldn't even wear for Halloween! Even when a model in a photoshoot looks "normal" or "natural," there is a huge amount of effort that goes into creating that perfect camera shot. There are usually at least five people (artists, actually) involved and working VERY hard—from hair to makeup, to clothing, to lighting, to actual camera operation.

Real life can never really look the way it does in a glossy photoshoot. But in real life, makeup can give us a sense of confidence. It can help us look more well-rested. It can make us look more alert, more engaged, more awake. This sharpness can actually help our true personality shine through. Instead of looking at a temporary blemish on our face, our audience is looking at the beautiful sparkle in our eyes or our gorgeous smile.

Have you ever had that friend who says, "you look tired." Even if you *are* tired, do you really want everyone around you *thinking* that? Worse yet, I've had weird acquaintances (notice I didn't say "friends") who have told me I look sick, when, in fact, I'm just not wearing any makeup. (I guess that's reason enough for me to pull out the brush!)

If I look too tired, who is going to trust me with a difficult task or responsibility? It's precisely in these situations that makeup has the power of helping me say, "I am in charge of my life. I am empowered. I can face the world head-on. Go ahead, try me."

Good makeup is about having your best foot forward, not about trying to convince people that you're something you're not. You don't have to wear makeup to a workout. You don't have to wear it while you relax on the beach. But, when you want to make a good first impression or give a strong presentation, I think makeup is very appropriate. While makeup isn't a neccesity, it's an opportunity to look and feel your best.

Savvy is Different...

There are so many brands, types, and styles of makeup, that it can be difficult to choose between them. In getting savvy about makeup, it requires patience to explore, study, practice, experiment, and perfect.

As a Master Esthetician and 30-year cosmetologist, I've pretty much tried every single brand of skin care, hair care, and cosmetic product. It's just what I do. That said, I've taken a greater and greater approach to natural solutions. While I've administered harsh chemical peels, toxic chemical injections, and assisted with painful aesthetic procedures, I've come to value a more natural philosophy. Our bodies were made to be well-cared-for by the things Mother Nature intended. Sure, there are pharmaceutical skin products that yield dramatic results, but at what cost?

I've witnessed so much irritation, pain, and self-mutilation for the cause of beauty, that it turns my stomach. There has to be a better way! The good news? There is...

This decade has seen a huge number of companies trying to be more responsible and create more eco-friendly, cruelty-free, non-synthetic options. What's funny is that these companies are suddenly trying to do what Young Living has done for nearly 30 years!

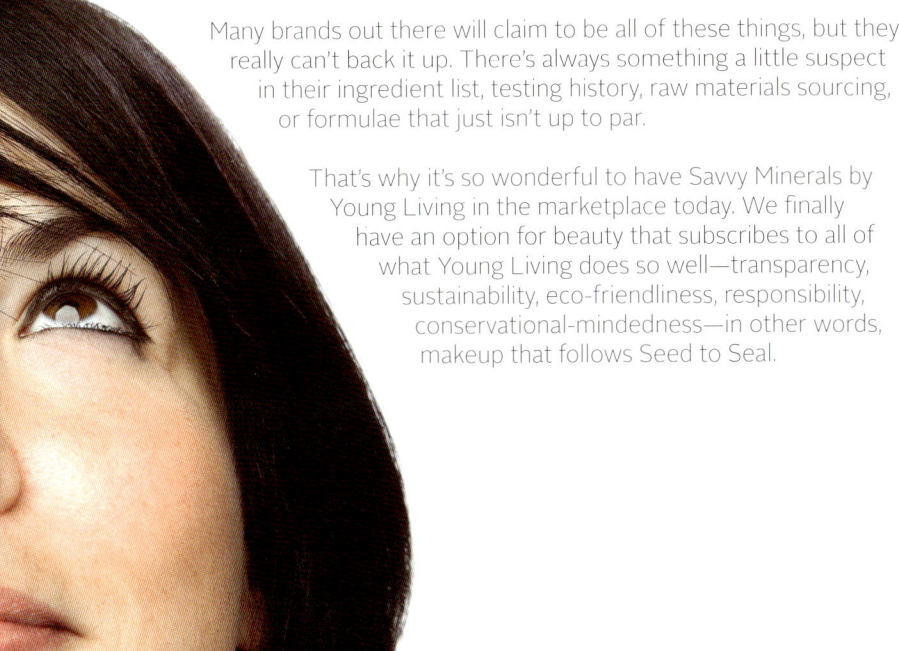

Many brands out there will claim to be all of these things, but they really can't back it up. There's always something a little suspect in their ingredient list, testing history, raw materials sourcing, or formulae that just isn't up to par.

That's why it's so wonderful to have Savvy Minerals by Young Living in the marketplace today. We finally have an option for beauty that subscribes to all of what Young Living does so well—transparency, sustainability, eco-friendliness, responsibility, conservational-mindedness—in other words, makeup that follows Seed to Seal.

A Clean Line for Clean Living

Completely Free Of:

 TOXINS

 BPA

 TALC

 PETROCHEMICALS

 BISMUTH

 CHEAP FILLERS

 PARABENS

 SYNTHETIC DYES

 PHTHALATES

 HEAVY METALS

 GLUTEN

 COAL TAR

 NYLON

 HARSH CHEMICALS

 ACRYLICS

 NANOPARTICLES

 POLYVINYLS

 SYNTHETIC FRAGRANCE

Plus: CRUELTY-FREE, VEGAN-FRIENDLY, KOSHER, & HALAL!

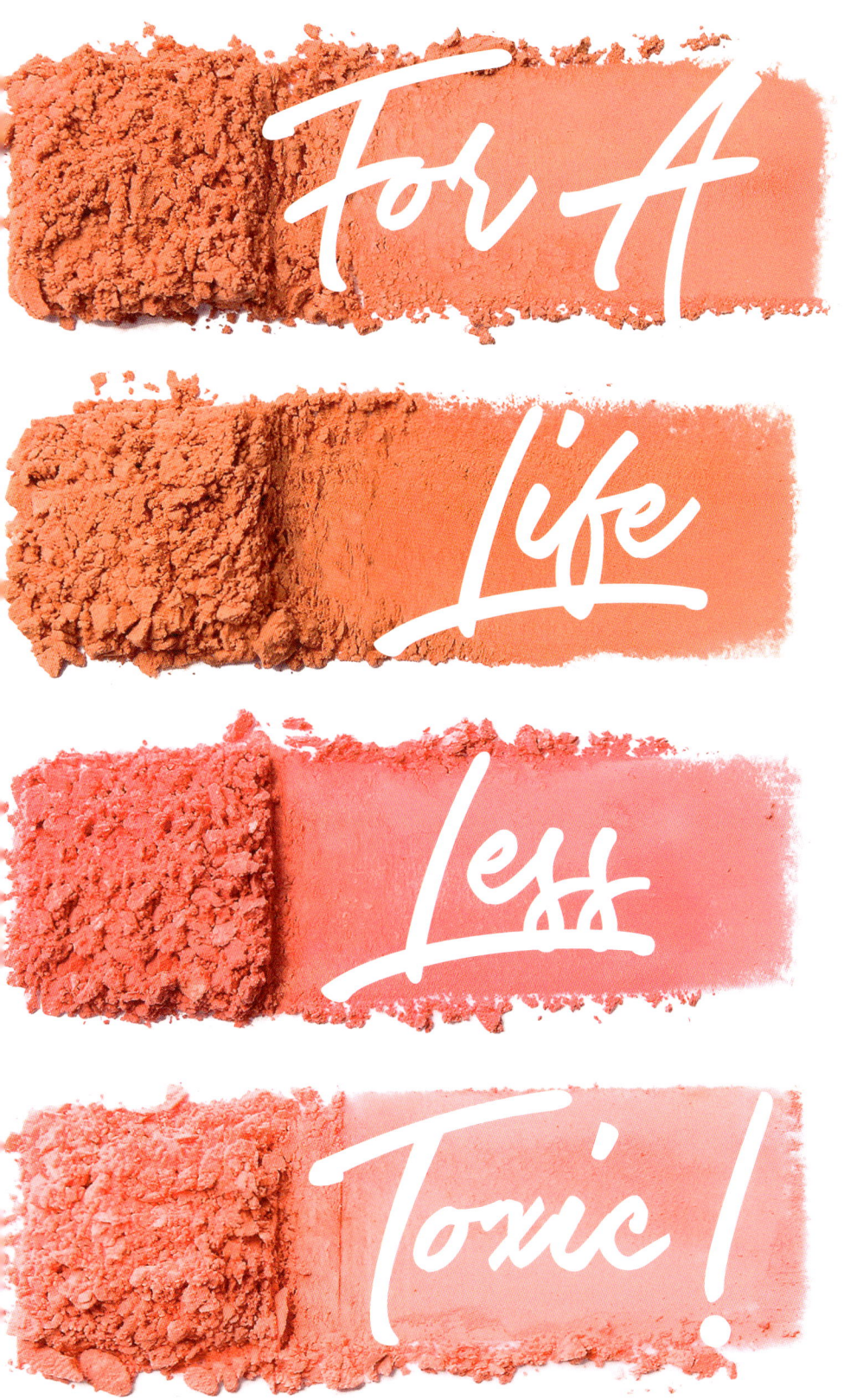

For A
Life
Less
Toxic!

The Levels of Makeup

So, let's talk. Makeup can be a wonderful thing. Once upon a time, say in the sixties, you could unapologetically take a heavy hand and draw a crayon line around your eyes and call it daily wear. Women wore wigs and wore enormous, thick false eyelashes—sometimes two pair at a time. (Think Austin Powers.) It was the Nancy Sinatra go-go boots (that were made for walkin') swingin' sixties and makeup was part of the party.

Times have changed a little, and we now go for a more natural look. We all want to look like we just woke up in this magically natural way, with a sparkle in our eye and a wide-awake look that seems ready to take on the world. We want to take what nature gave us and make it just a little better.

I break it down into what I call *Levels of Makeup*. Don't get me wrong, every one of these levels is appropriate. I just don't want you looking like a rodeo clown, unless you truly are going to the rodeo and you're actually *getting paid* to be a *clown*!

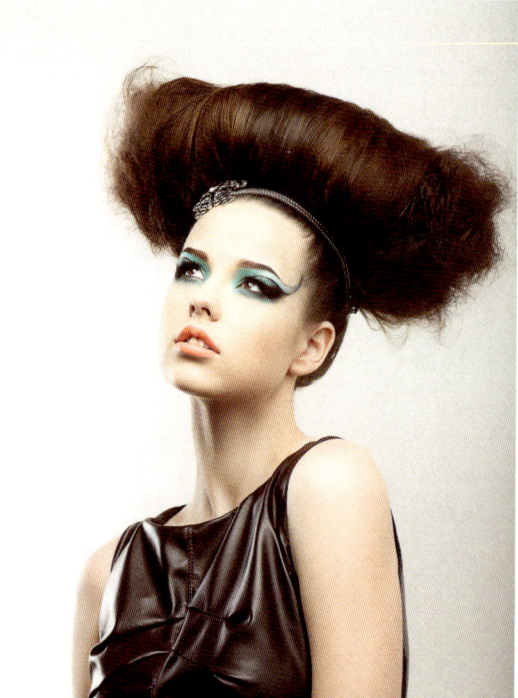

CAUTION!
Not recommended
as an everyday look...

DEFINING / ENHANCING / EMBOLDENING

At this level, you are taking the wonderful features that Mother Nature has given you and making them more obvious. You're making your brows have sharper starting and ending points. You're enhancing the line of your lips and smoothing them over with a little gloss and barely-there color.

MASKING / CONCEALING

This is where you take the parts of your appearance that aren't your favorite—perhaps the dark circles under your eyes, the broken capillaries, pimples, permanent or transient blemishes, blackheads—and finding ways to mask them. They are still there. They're just not so obvious.

MAGNIFYING

This is the level you project when you are confident, brave, and have that unapologetic application of your favorite lipstick. It may be a little more outré. It may be more loud and obvious. In other words, at this level of makeup, you're not trying so hard to look like you're not wearing makeup. You know that people know you are wearing it, and it's perfectly fine. At this level, don't be surprised when people say "I love your makeup!" You take it as a compliment, because that's your effort being recognized.

ALTERING

This level of makeup goes beyond the natural. Some people adopt this philosophy on a daily basis, but it takes a good deal of effort. This is where you are contouring, wearing multiple levels of foundation, and are using those varying degrees to actually alter how the light captures your features. For most of us, this is reserved for events or for professional or nearly-professional photography—in a studio or controlled setting. This is the kind of makeup you wear to your wedding, your daughter's wedding, for a photoshoot, or perhaps a high-profile evening event.

TRANSFORMING

Usually we reserve this for Halloween, but we might have other occasions that call for more drastic measures. This may be a television appearance, a stage appearance, or participation in an art piece. Make no mistake. Sometimes you'll see this behind a fast-food counter and wonder if it's Halloween and you somehow forgot. But, for the most part, we hit this level once or twice a year at most!

The Basic Philosophy

If you didn't grow up around a lot of makeup, or if you've set it aside while focusing on other things, there's really no right way to do it. The truth is, every woman is different. Every woman has a different comfort level when she puts something on her face. What feels good, natural, and easy for you may not be to someone else and vice-versa. As you examine your caboodle, don't think of *right* or *wrong*. Think of what works for you, what feels safe on your skin, and what makes you feel confident.

GROWING

Most of us first experienced makeup through our mothers and grandmothers. We then decided to experiment by goofing around with our friends. We may have even gone to a makeup counter for a "makeover" when were still teens just to learn how to apply a certain brand, product, color, or makeup type. The important thing about makeup is that we have an attitude of growing. We have to be willing to learn something new.

LEARNING

That said, we learn by applying and practicing. The first time we put on mascara with a wand, we struggle first with blinking and then with having thick, pasty black crusty cake on our eyes all day. We do it all for the sake of beauty.

EXPLORING

The only way we learn something new is by exploring. We have to be willing to try different colors, different application techniques, different preparation products, and different application tools. All of this takes time and means that we don't get down on ourselves or feel embarrassed when we make mistakes. The world of makeup at the highest levels is still chock-full of makeup missteps. So what? If you have an off time of it, just crack it up to exeprience!

CREATING

Each of us has an inner muse. We all have potential to be creative. That's what makeup is all about. Every time you hear about one set of rules, the next thing you know, all the top players are breaking them! The world of makeup is a constantly evolving, ever-changing stage—and that's a good thing!

EXPERIMENTING

So go ahead. Be daring. Be bold. Experiment. Try something new every weekend of the month, until you find exactly what you like.

DISCOVERING

As you unleash your inner makeup maven, catalog what you learn. Commit your favorite techniques, products, colors, and shades to paper or memory. When it comes to getting acquainted with the whole Savvy line, I recommend having a party with like-minded friends who just want to explore the possibilities. Get your girlfriends together, gather your makeup, share what you love most, and learn why other people have a favorite. In short, awaken your inner child and give yourself permission to have play time! Hey, I say go heavy on the Inner Child™ in the diffuser and enjoy!

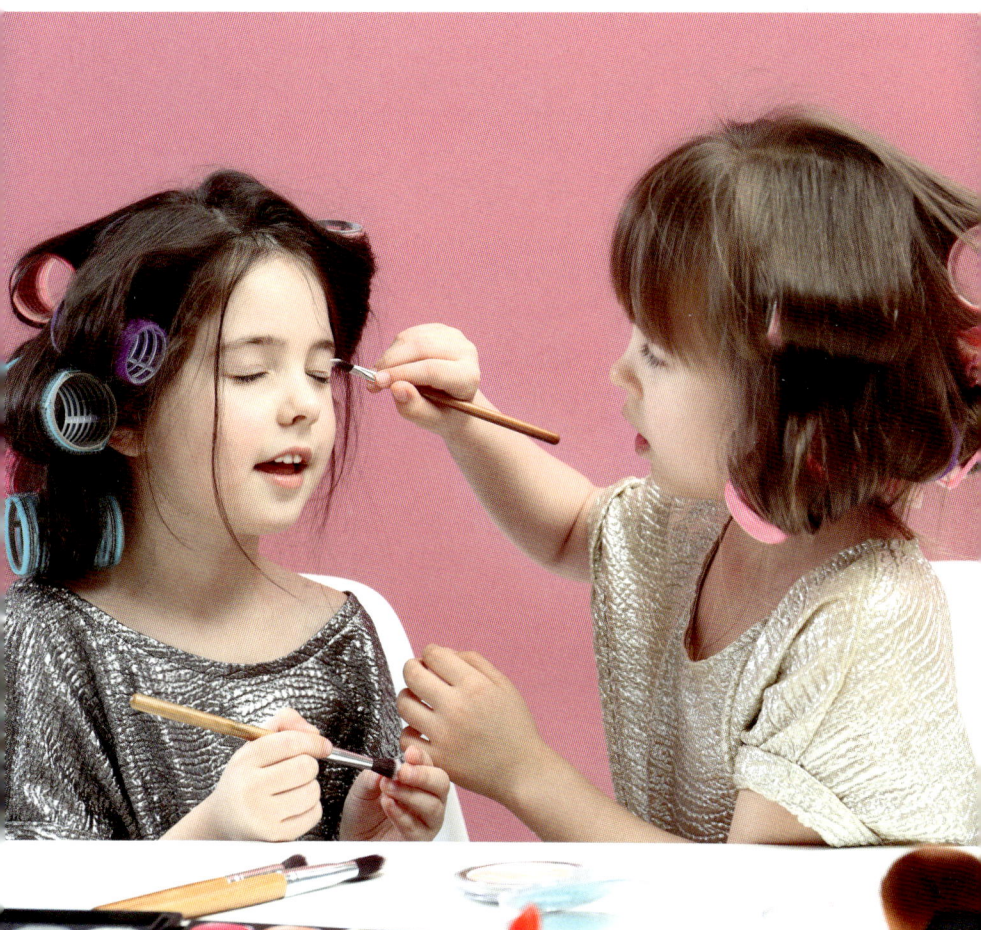

A Clean Canvas

START CLEAN

So you have to start with a clean slate. If you wipe your face after cleaning with a towel and there is still makeup on it, chances are, you're not cleaning properly.

There are basically three types of cleansers for three skin types:

Cream = Dry Skin
Gel = Oily Skin
Milk = Ultra-sensitive Skin

Avoid washing with hot water. While it may *feel* spa-like and rejuvenating, it can cause broken capillaries—a particularly common problem for those of us over a certain age. Ultra-cold water can cause similar issues, so the best temperature to use when you lather is lukewarm.

Be gentle. Always use gentle, circular, upward motions as you apply cleanser to your entire face and neck. Never pull down on your skin, scrub aggressively, or scratch at it.

Thanks to Young Living's new Seedlings® line, you can use the same toxin-free gentle wipes on your face that you would on a baby's bottom! These are great for removing your waterproof makeup. Also, Life Science Publishing's *DIY: Beauty* has a wonderful recipe for natural, do-it-yourself makeup wipes.

ART® Gentle Cleanser is good for all skin types and can be your go-to option for cleansing. Even if you cleanse twice, this product won't overdry your skin.

If you have particularly heavy, waterproof mascara, try a little V-6® on a cotton ball or pad and gently massage off your eye makeup without pulling on the lashes. Try gently rolling back and forth over them. This may take a few gentle swipes.

If you're oily and not particularly sensitive, try Orange Blossam Facial Wash. If you're acneic, I recommend Satin Facial Scrub™, Mint.

Finish out your cleaning regimen with ART® Refreshing Toner. It gently helps to tighten pores after they open up from cleaning.

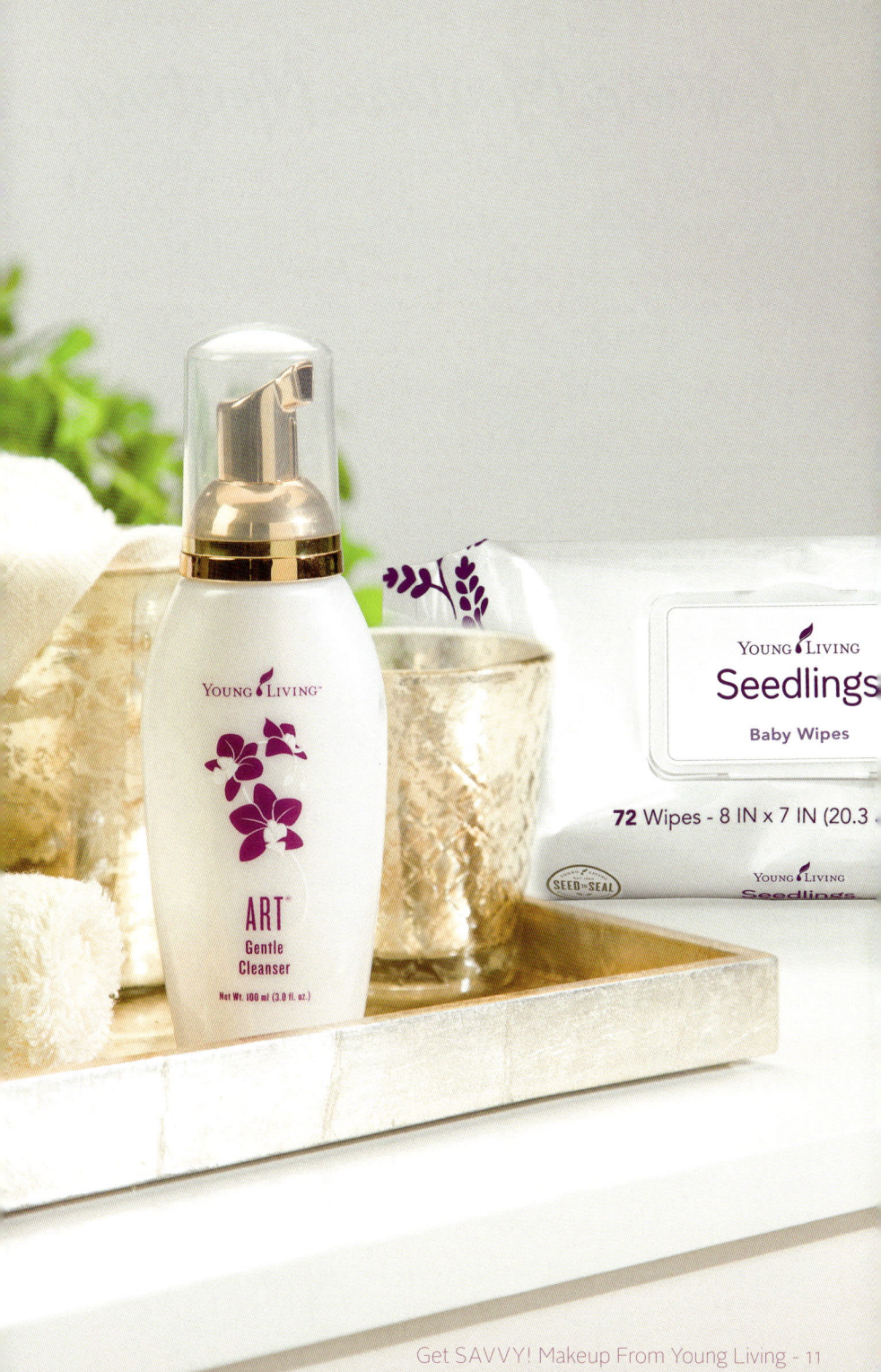

YOUNG LIVING™

ART®
Gentle
Cleanser

Net Wt. 100 ml (3.0 fl. oz.)

YOUNG LIVING
Seedlings
BABY WIPES

72 Wipes - 8 IN x 7 IN (20.3

SEED TO SEAL

YOUNG LIVING
Seedlings

Moisture. Moisture. Moisture.

Nothing is more important in maintaining a youthful appearance like moisture. Different types of skin require a different level of moisture. Fortunately, Young Living has created two basic types that really get the job done without causing breakouts:

- ART® Intensive Moisturizer (Creme Masque)
- ART® Light Moisturizer

Beyond moisture, one of the best ways to get a real balanced complexion is with Sheerlumé. This proprietary blend from Young Living helps you visibly brighten and balance. The great news is that you can use it in conjunction with either of the two moisturizers. It also works well with oily, dry, or combination skin.

PREPARING

The world's top makeup artists spend up to an hour preparing their clients' skin before they ever touch it with makeup. They take care of skin health first, preparing it so that everything can go on smoothly and evenly. Then they proceed to camouflage, cover, shape, color, and set.

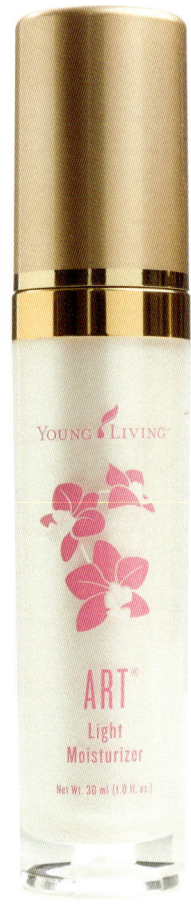

The same should be true for any of us. We may not have an hour, but we can certainly take our 15 minutes of cleaning and treating before we go to bed, 15 minutes of care when we wake up, and 5-10 minutes for our makeup. Beautiful, healthy skin is worth 35 minutes a day, right? And, if you're ready to learn all the ways that Young Living's beauty line can work to your full advantage, I recommend attending Young Living's *Beauty School*. It's a wonderful boot camp for anyone who wants to brush up on their skills!

YOUNG LIVING
DRY SKIN SERUM
ESSENTIAL BEAUTY
Net 0.5 fl. oz. (15 ml)
YOUNG LIVING
WOLFBERRY
EYE CREAM
Net WT 0.5 oz. (14.1 g)
YOUNG LIVING
SANDALWOOD
MOISTURE CREAM
Net Wt. 4 oz. (113 g)
YOUNG LIVING
A·R·T
BEAUTY MASQUE
SOOTHING FACIAL MASQUE
WITH ORCHID PETALS & ESSENTIAL OILS
CONTENTS: 8 MASQUES
Mary Young

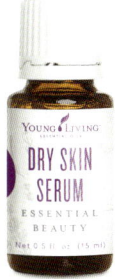

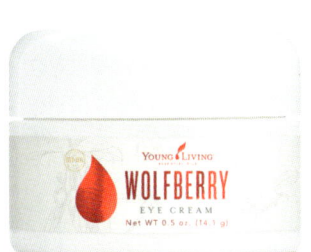

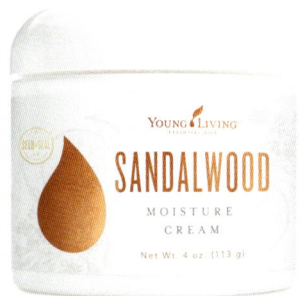

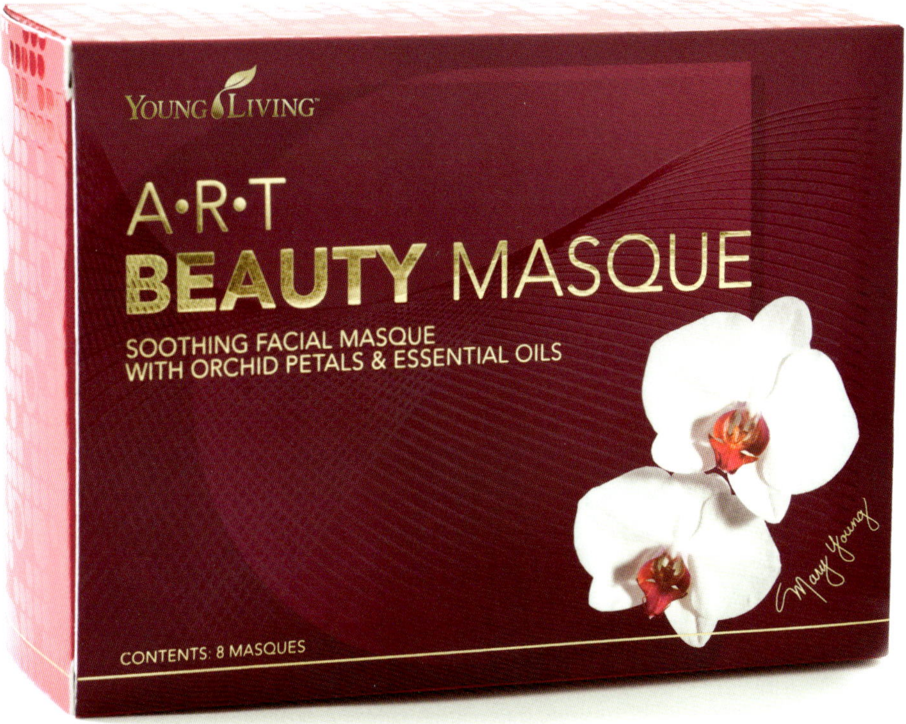

Balance & Protection

One of the biggest causes of aging is sun damage. From fine lines, to wrinkles, to actinic keratosis, to freckles and liver spots, the sun has a way of doing more harm than good. Luckily, Young Living has provided a really good solution in the form of Mineral Sunscreen Lotion.

As someone who has worked for (and with) high-end dermatologists, esthetic surgeons/nurse practitioners, and the largest medical day spa group west of the Mississippi, I can tell you that barrier sunscreen makes all the difference. Anyone, who's anyone, will tell you that.

While Young Living's Mineral Sunscreen Lotion is only rated 10 SPF, it still has many advantages. It has UVA/UVB, broad spectrum protection. It goes on smooth and creamy, it's non-nano, and it's free from all the synthetics and toxins you'll usually find in other brands.

What I love about it, is that I can put it on over Sheerlumé, and it gives me not only added moisture but also a "brightened" sheen that floats on top of my skin. I can then apply mineral makeup over the top and have the added benefit of the natural mineral reflection that makes me feel protected.

Now, I wouldn't spend all day at the beach tanning in it, but it does what I need for a natural all-day protection. Also, I tend to be dry, so the emollient factor in this works just fine. For those with acneic or oily skin, this may not be the best fit.

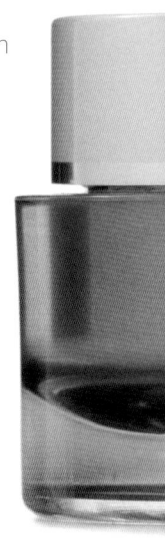

Benefits:
- Broad-spectrum SPF 10 sunscreen protection
- Blocks UVA and UVB rays
- Water resistant and sweat proof for 80 minutes
- Helps prevent sunburns
- Smooths easily onto skin and won't leave a white residue
- Made with naturally derived plant- & mineral-based ingredients
- Formulated for those with sensitive skin
- Dermatologist tested and hypoallergenic
- Formulated without UV chemical absorbers, parabens, phthalates, petrochemicals, animal-derived ingredients, synthetic preservatives, synthetics fragrances, or synthetic dyes

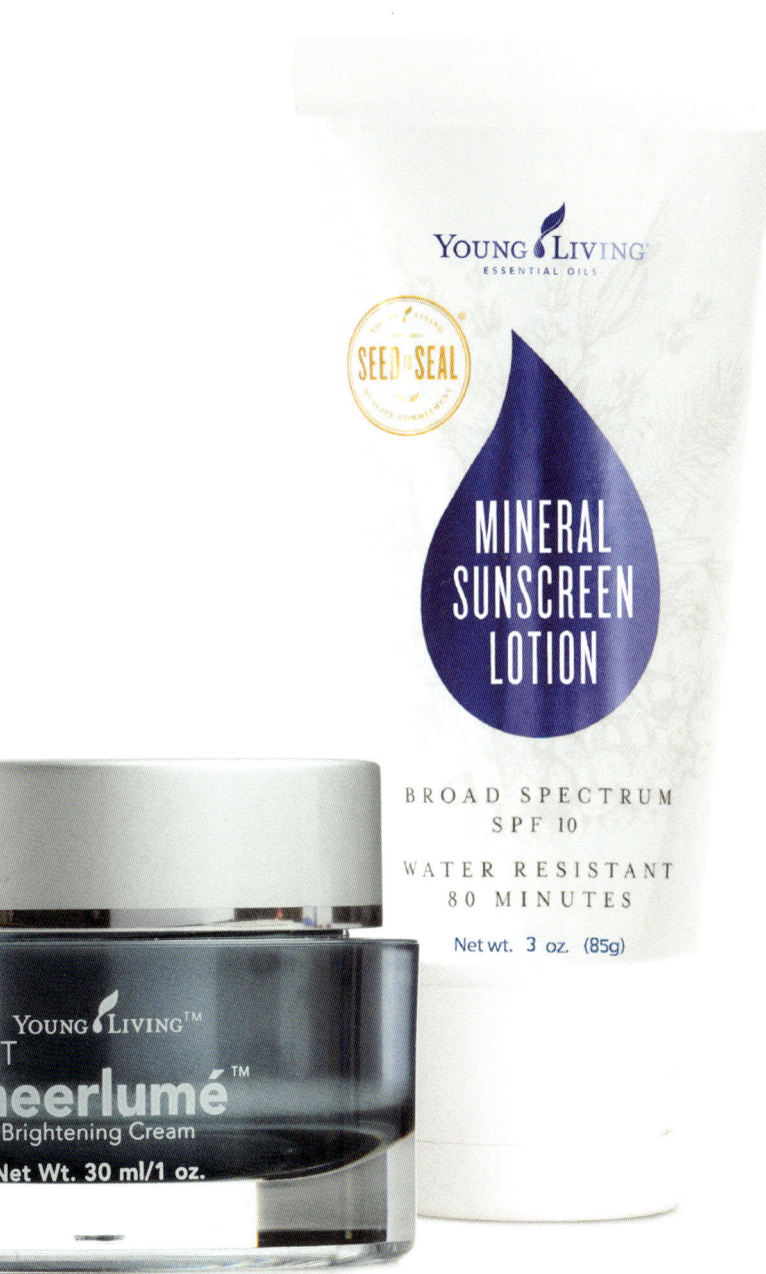

Treat it Right

The best time to treat your skin is right when you've cleaned it. This is the best time to treat your broken capillaries, your acne, blackheads, redness, pores, and other conditions. Here are some guidelines for using essential oils to combat your everyday skin issues...

BROKEN CAPILLARIES =
1) ART® Renewal Serum, Amoressence™†
2) Add three drops of any of the following to 1/2 teaspoon of ART® Light Moisturizer: Helichrysum, Geranium, Rose, Roman Chamomile, German Chamomile, Frankincense, Lavender

ACNE =
1) ART® Renewal Serum, Amoressence™†
2) Add three drops of any of the following to 1/2 teaspoon of ART® Light Moisturizer: Tea Tree, Geranium, Vetiver, Sandalwood, Lavender, German Chaomile, Cedarwood, Orange, Neroli

BLACKHEADS =
1) ART® Renewal Serum, Amoressence™†
2) Add three drops of any of the following to 1/2 teaspoon of ART® Light Moisturizer: Tea Tree, Lavender, Eucalyptus, Lemon, Juniper, Clary Sage, Lemongrass*

REDNESS =
1) ART® Renewal Serum, Amoressence™†
2) Add three drops of any of the following to 1/2 teaspoon of ART® Light Moisturizer: Tea Tree, Lavender, Eucalyptus, Geranium, Chamomile, Rose, Rosemary*, Thyme*

PORES =
ART® Refreshing Toner, ART® Beauty Mask, ART® Creme Masque

INFLAMED, DRY, ITCHY, OR PATCHY =
1) ART® Beauty Mask, ART® Creme Masque
2) Add three drops of any of the following to 1/2 teaspoon of ART® Light Moisturizer: Roman Chamomile, Geranium, Juniper, Sandalwood, Rose, Lavender

*Can be considered a "hot" oil. Use only in dilution of at least 1 to 4
† Available only at *Young Living Beauty School*

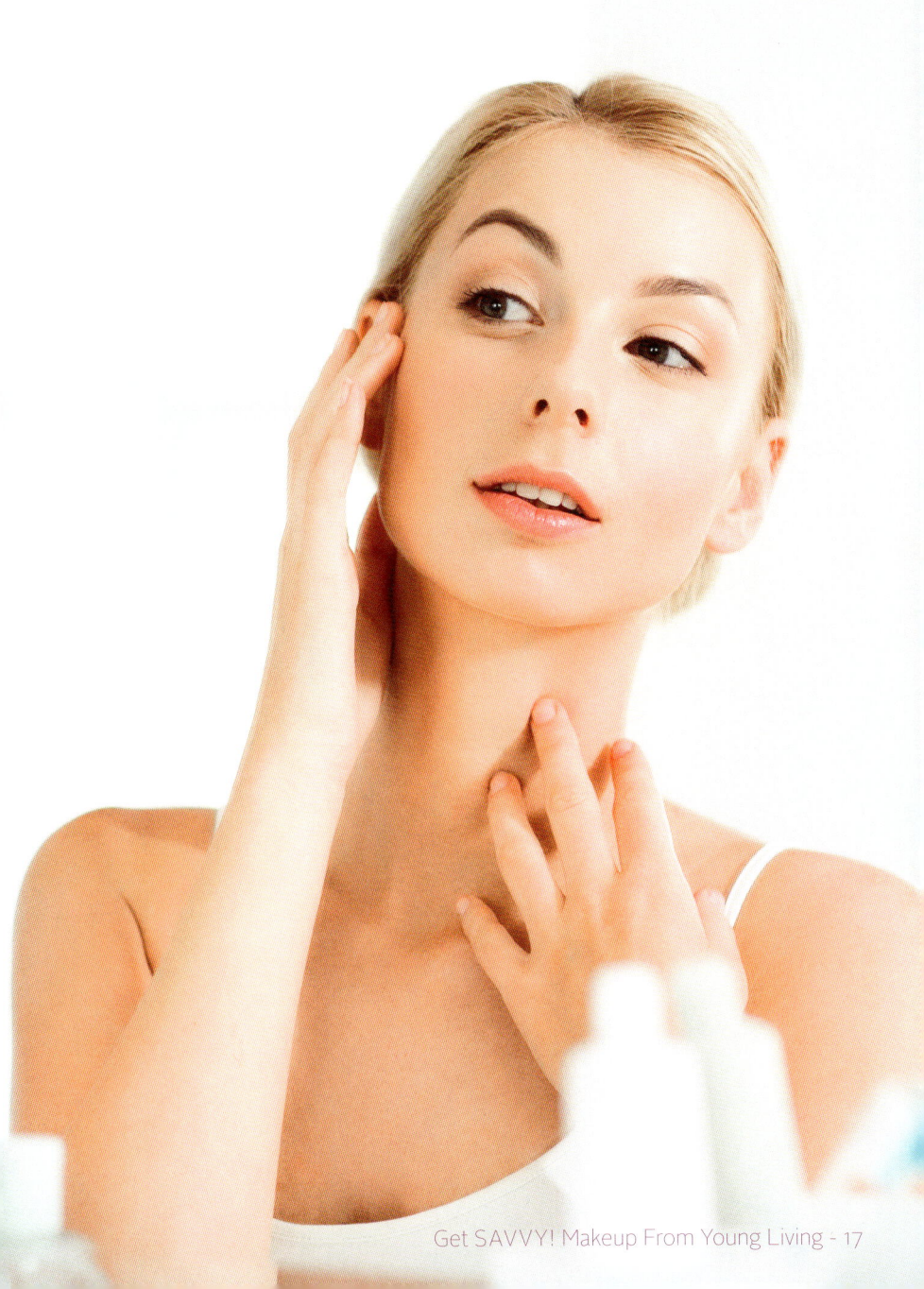

Makeup is what you *make up*. It's not what you *have* to do or *should* do. There isn't *one right way* to make up a face. Makeup is about creativity, self-determination, empowerment, grace, and satisfaction. The only *right* makeup is the one that is *free of toxins*—the kind you apply *from your* own *world-view*, expressive of your *personality*, and reflective of your *soul*.

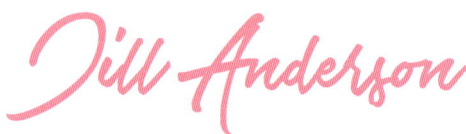

BE BRAVE

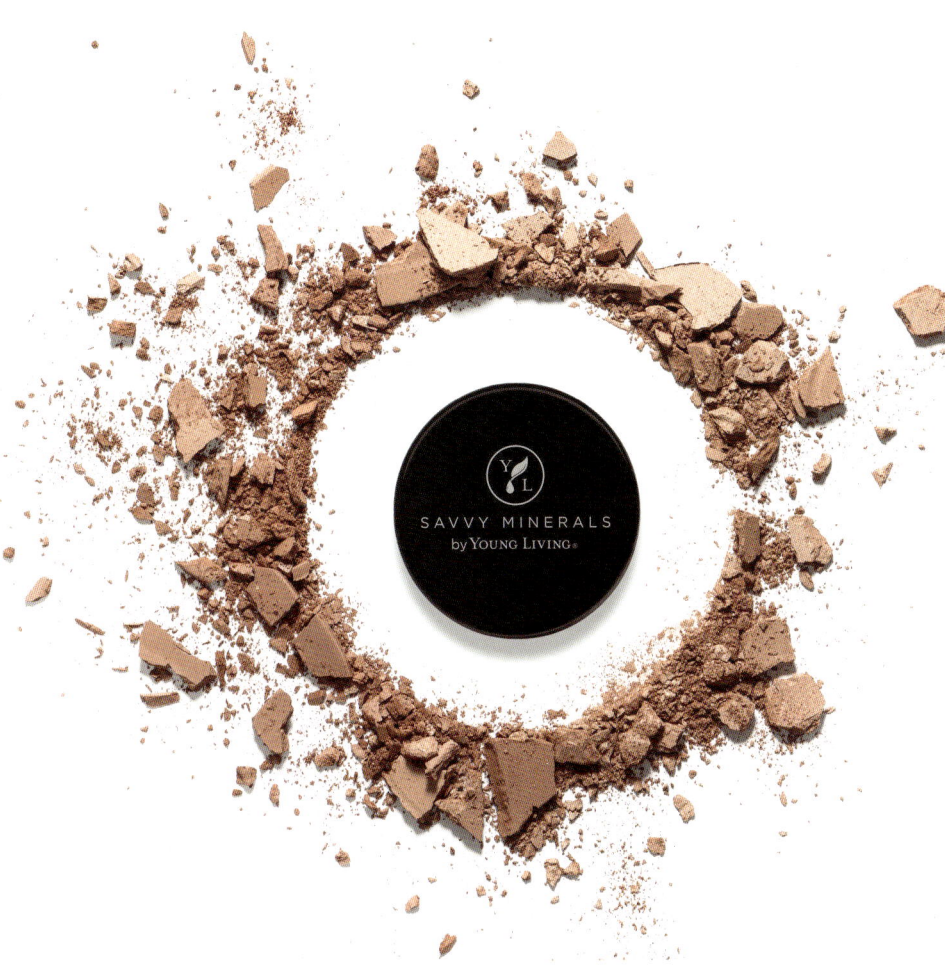

GET READY TO DITCH & SWITCH

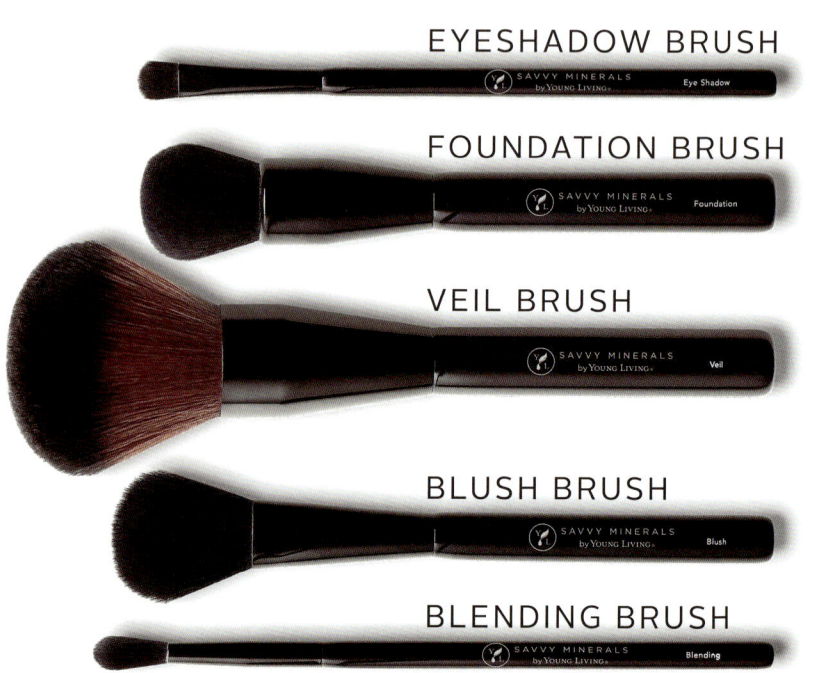

EYESHADOW BRUSH

FOUNDATION BRUSH

VEIL BRUSH

BLUSH BRUSH

BLENDING BRUSH

S A V V Y   B R U S H E S

Compared to many of the brushes in high-end retail stores and makeup counters, this set of five high-quality brushes can really be a great deal—especially when you consider wholesale pricing for members, PV (Personal Volume), and Essential Rewards. The whole design and sourcing of these brushes is for working optimally with the Savvy Mineral line—so you get the right amount on your brush every time! Plus, you get the handy carrying case that advertises for you every time you pull it out of your purse for touch-ups!

FOUNDATION BRUSH
May be used to apply foundation or bronzer.

EYESHADOW BRUSH
Great for eyeshadow application & even brow definition.

BLUSH BRUSH
Perfect for applying blush or bronzer.

BLENDING BRUSH
Good for contouring, blending in eyeshadow, or taking the edge off of an over-application or heavy spot.

VEIL BRUSH
This is perfect for that perfect, final finish with Diamond Dust Veil finishing powder.

MISTING SPRAY

This specially-formulated Misting Spray helps you to control the application, pigment, and even distribution of the particles. Naturally-derived to help keep the line safe and toxin-free. Use it to concentrate color on brushes before applying.

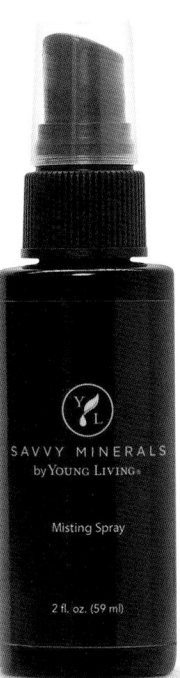

CONTOUR BRUSH
Contour, add blush, or work your bronzer.

BRONZER BRUSH
Use the angle to contour or add blush.

CONCEALER BRUSH
Great for stippling smaller areas, applying beneath the eyes & fixing more obvious trouble spots.

EYEBROW BRUSH
Comb, shape, & tame the brows while applying brow filler.

EYELINER BRUSH
Great for creating tight, precise, & fine lines.

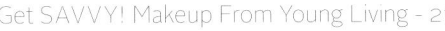

FOUNDATION

This is basis of any truly effective makeup. With a buildable formula, you'll be able to apply light to heavy with a few simple layers. Prepare to feel flawless all day with a soft, satin finish.

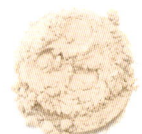 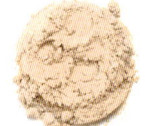 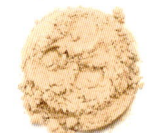

WARM No.1   WARM No.2   WARM No.3

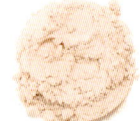 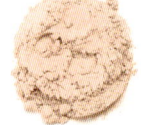 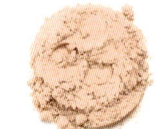

COOL No.1   COOL No.2   COOL No.3

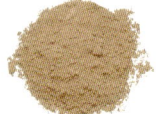 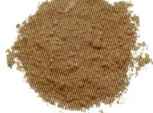 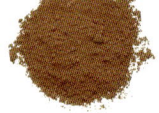 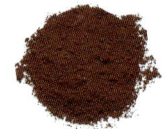

DARK No.1   DARK No.2   DARK No.3   DARK No.4

SUMMER LOVED   CROWNED ALL OVER

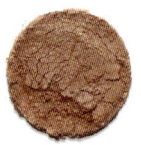 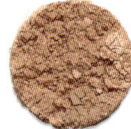

BRONZER

It doesn't take much of Savvy Minerals Bronzer to get a soft, sun-kissed look. The added shine gives you a pearlescent finish that blends well with your foundation. If you want a more matte feel, try using a darker foundation in its place. Or, mix a darker foundation with your favorite of the two bronzers for the perfect sun-touched shade.

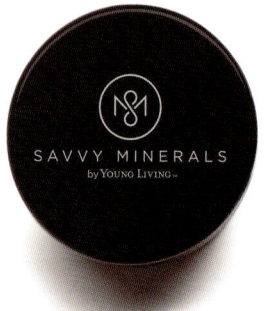

BLUSH

Flawless skin looks great, until it's flat and all-one-color. Thanks to Savvy Minerals Blush, three gorgeous shades help you add that natural flush to your cheeks. No need to feel stark and all-one-color. The colors build naturally and you can add touch-ups throughout the day.

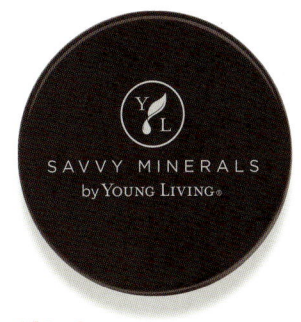

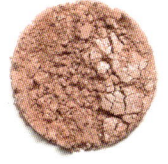 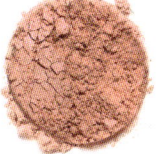 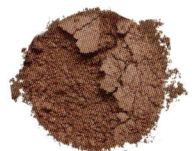

I DO BELIEVE YOU'RE BLUSHIN'   SMASHING   PASSIONATE

EYESHADOW

This clean palette of Savvy Minerals Eyeshadow offers a nice high-to-low range of shading through natural, rich pigments. The variety makes it easy to create a range of looks for highlighting and lowlighting in living color. The formula allows you to build, but stays colorfast all day long. The blendability makes it so you can go from desk to dinner (or daywear to nightwear) with a few simple brushstrokes.

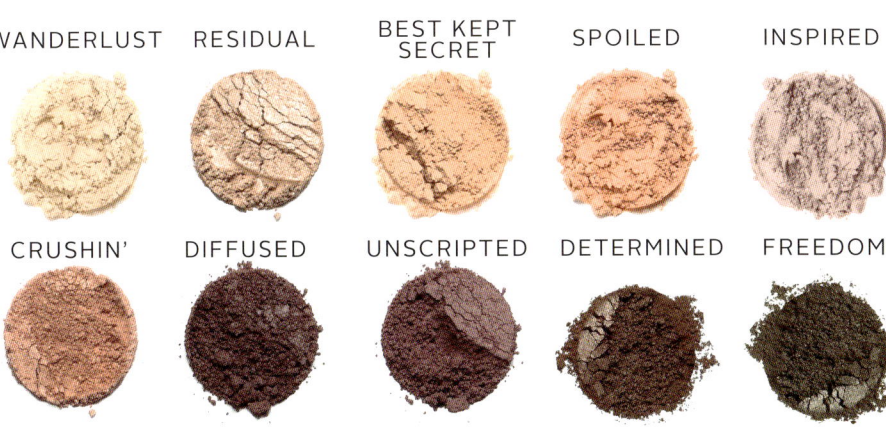

WANDERLUST   RESIDUAL   BEST KEPT SECRET   SPOILED   INSPIRED

CRUSHIN'   DIFFUSED   UNSCRIPTED   DETERMINED   FREEDOM

EYELINER

JET SETTER

The eyes come alive with two great shades of liner. Multitasker actually doubles as an eyebrow filler, triples as an eyeshadow. Jet Setter works to create subtle or high-impact eyes. With a little practice, either one can create sultry, smoky, cat, Egyptian, or almond eyes. Mix the two for even greater versatility.

MULTITASKER

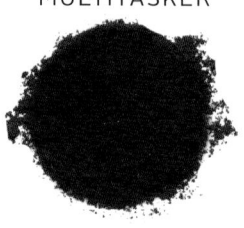

MASCARA

Nothing conditions and supports your own ability to produce long, healthy lashes like Young Living Lavender essential oil. That's why it's such a unique feature in this formula. Smudge-free and long-lasting, you'll love knowing that you're supporting healthy lashes, while showcasing them. The formula builds with clumping. Best of all, it doesn't have the usual culprits that all other mascara brands have. Putting a natural product next to your eyes is a must!

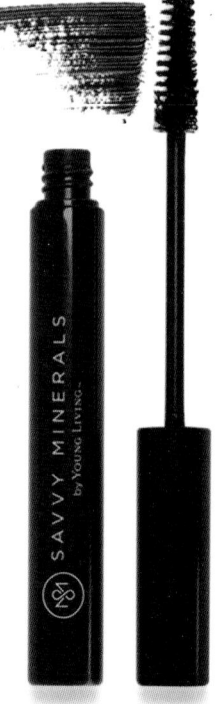

FINISHING/SETTING POWDER

Depending on your skin type (how much moisture your skin holds), you might opt for this translucent powder. It absorbs oil and creates a luminous finish as it sets your look. Some people may even opt to use it alone as super sheer balancer/evener. It may potentially highlight your color slightly, so keep that in mind when you choose your foundation color(s). It comes singularly in Diamond Dust, so remember to run it down the neckline and blend across the shoulders and/or collarbone, if you're taking photos.

For mature clients, I recommend only using this in the T-zone, nose, and chinline. You want to steer clear of powdering areas that could cake into fine lines throughout the day.

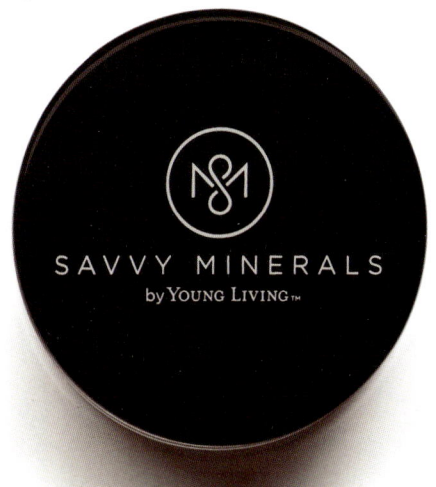

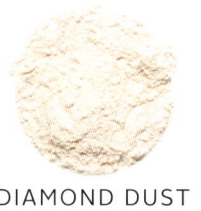

DIAMOND DUST

LIPSTICK *

So you may not be able to match every color of every blouse in your closet, but you can definitely create a natural, beautiful, flattering shade. The neutral tones look great on a wide range of skin types. As always, for whiter teeth, choose a cooler color with more bluish or berry undertones.

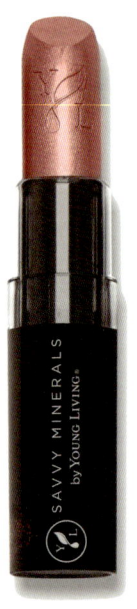 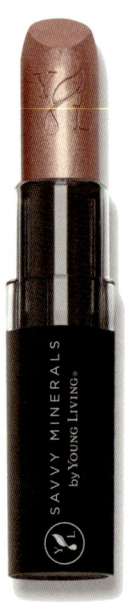 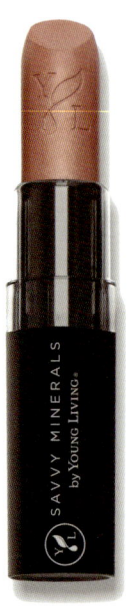 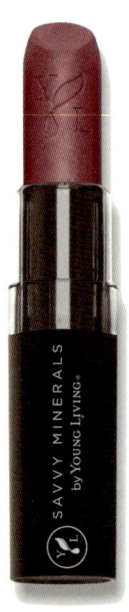 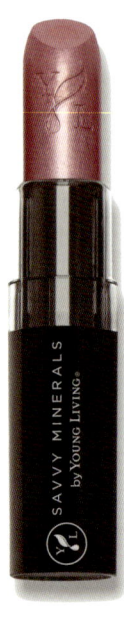

L I P G L O S S *

Conditioning your lips is every bit as important as the color you put on them. The beauty of Savvy Minerals Lipgloss is the soothing, softening you experience as you apply tint, color, and shine to your lips. Deepen the color by adding more than one coat. It's great for sheer to medium color. The colors have great depth and dimension, while still staying flatteringly neutral.

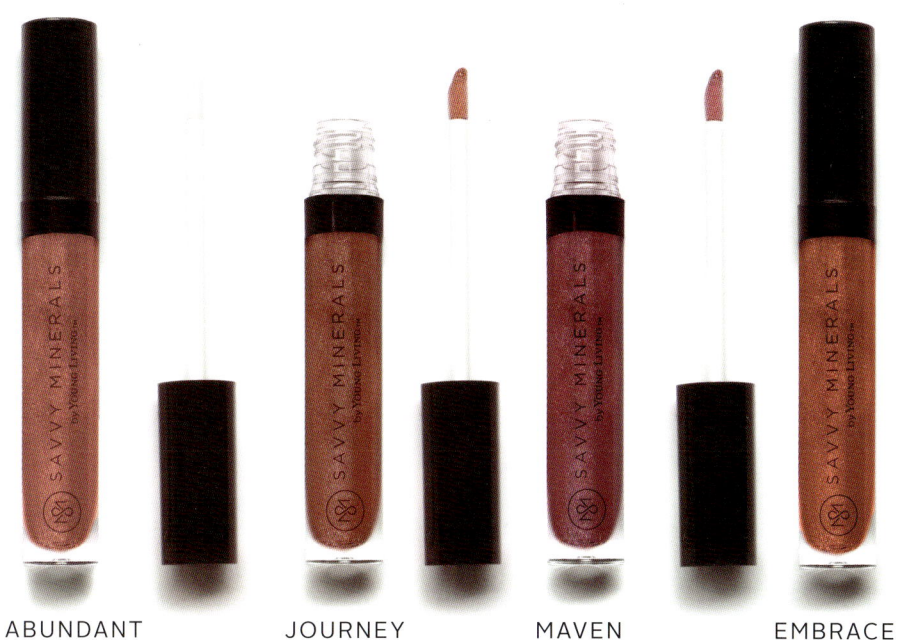

ABUNDANT   JOURNEY   MAVEN   EMBRACE

• The only Savvy Mineral products that aren't fully vegan, due to the use of natural beeswax.

The Process - From Start...

START CLEAN   ADD MOISTURE   TREAT & PREPARE

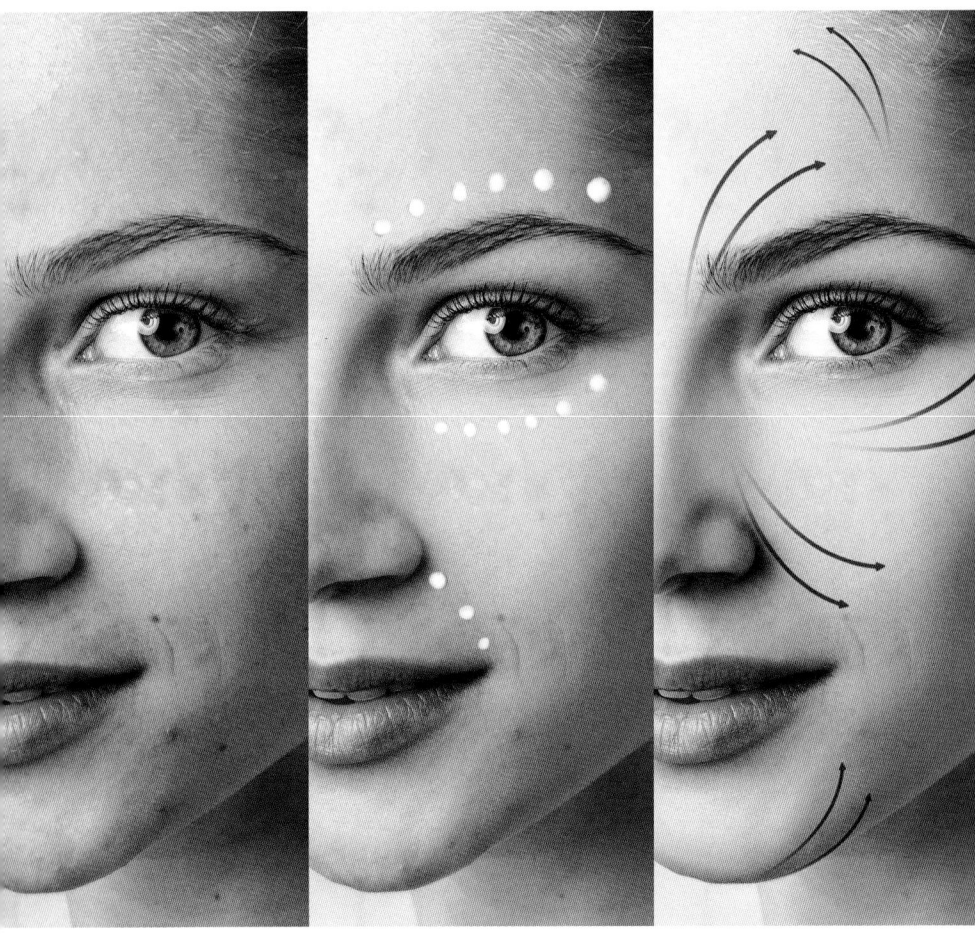

...to Finish!

PROTECT &
CONDITION

CONCEAL,
STIPPLE, &
CONTOUR

BLEND, DETAIL
EYES & BROWS,
& VEIL FINISH

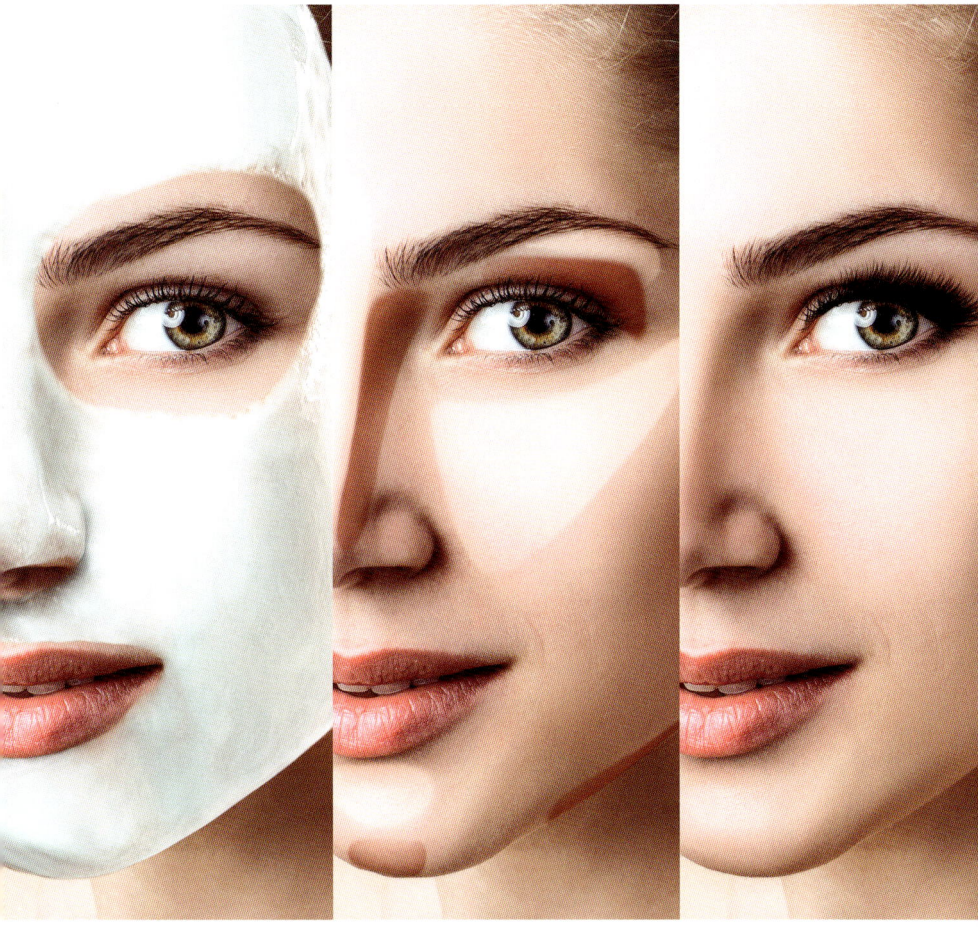

Face Facts

I said before that every face is different. It's absolutely true. Being unique is a good thing. No, really. The great news is that you're never really alone. Someone out there has a face similar in basic shape to yours, and makeup artists around the world have catalogued their best tips and tricks for making each face type shine (and I'm not talking oil or glitter).

We generally all fall into one of the following nine categories. The shapes speak for themselves.

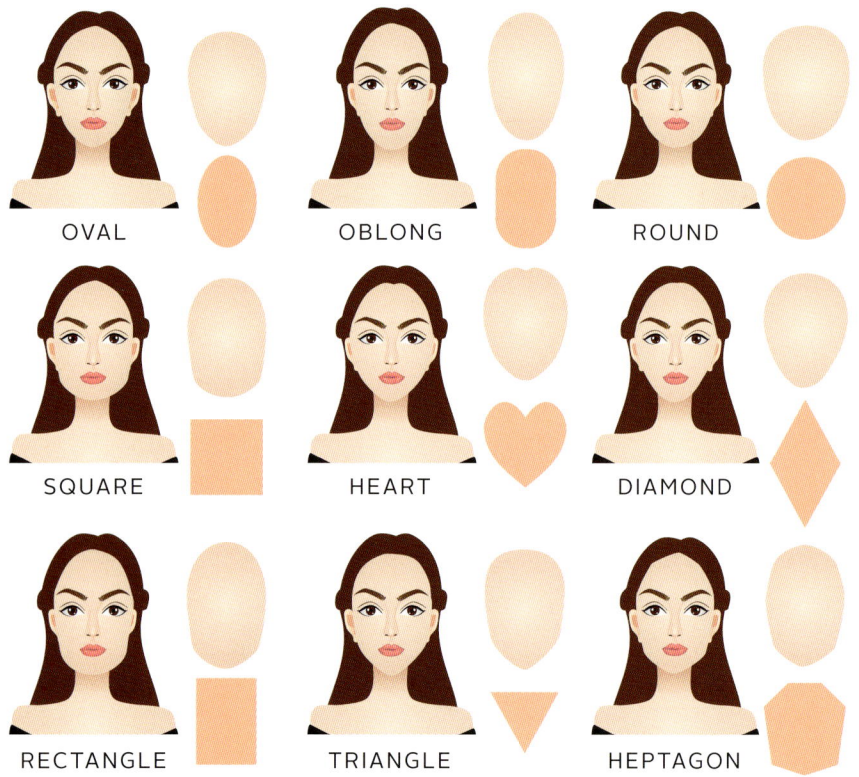

OVAL   OBLONG   ROUND

SQUARE   HEART   DIAMOND

RECTANGLE   TRIANGLE   HEPTAGON

Thanks to the Renaissance masters, we have learned that lighter color in a painting comes into the foreground, while dark colors recede. The same is true for maximizing and minimizing areas of the face. That's why you'll hear a lot of makeup artists for the Savvy line focusing so much on contouring. They are trying to help you make the most of your own personal face shape.

Now, this can be overwhelming for those who are just beginners, so keep it in mind, but don't let it discourage you, if it takes practice to get the hang of it.

With a little help from Kim K and her sisters, this makeup technique has received a lot of attention. I always offer it as a guideline, but remember one thing. Sonia Kashuk, Cindy Crawford, and Kevin Aucoin said to leave contouring in the studio with photoshoot artists where it belongs. If you're game, there are many YouTube videos that detail how to do it best.

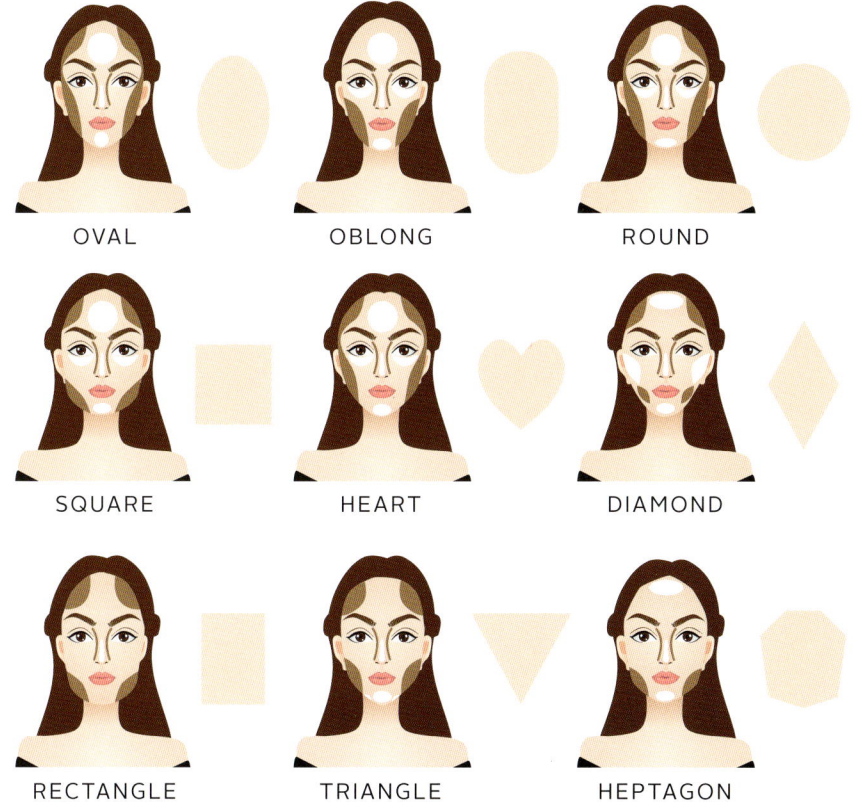

OVAL   OBLONG   ROUND

SQUARE   HEART   DIAMOND

RECTANGLE   TRIANGLE   HEPTAGON

Eye Facts

Let's talk about your eyes. After all, they can often do the talking for you! They are the windows to your soul and have the power to speak volumes. Generally, we take the eyes we are given and play them up. Here's how:

Almond eyes are very versatile and make up well with a full wash of color on the lash lid, a medium tone worn in the crease, and a dark color next to the lash line.

Downturned (or Droopy) eyes need a little dark color on the outer top lash line. Any eyeliner should focus on wings that go upward to counter the downturn.

Upturned eyes can use dark colors in the crease and liner that extends from the bottom middle to the outer edge.

Close-Set eyes need medium to dark shadow on outer third of the eylid to draw the shape outward.

Wide-Set eyes need look best by focusing color on the inner part of eyelids and avoiding too much definition on the outer corners.

Round eyes look best with a medium to dark shadow on the outer third of the lid. Try not to line the bottom part of the eye, because this will accentuate the roundness.

Protruding eyes need a little wash of medium color all across the top lid. Don't apply in the crease, since this will only accentuate the protrusion.

Hooded eyes need a greater focus on the lash line. Try a medium tone just above the crease to help soften teh browbone. Stay away from really light colors, or they'll accentuate the fleshy lid.

Monolid eyes need emphasis on the lash line and outer corner. Don't try to draw creases, if you're trying to look natural.

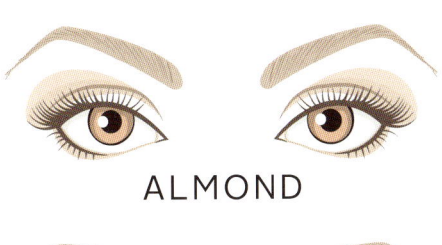

ALMOND

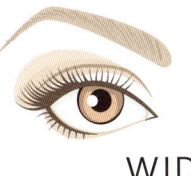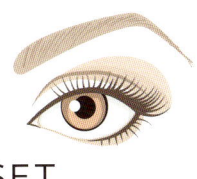

WIDE-SET

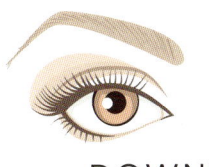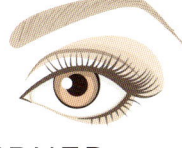

DOWNTURNED

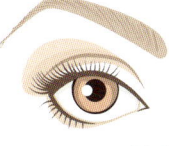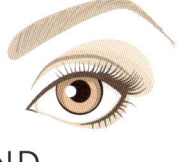

ROUND

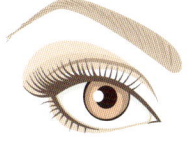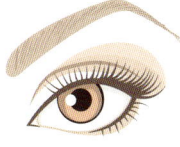

UPTURNED

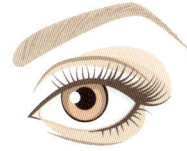

PROTRUDING

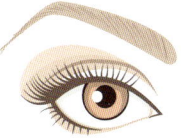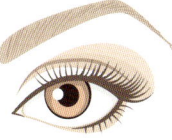

CLOSE-SET

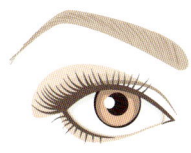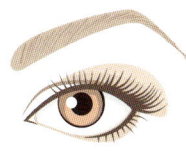

HOODED

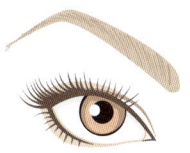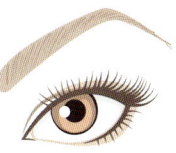

MONOLID

Eyebrow Facts

Your brows are responsible for a huge percentage of your facial expressions. Without them, our faces are cold, lonely plains—like the Russian Tundra.

If you tweeze, be careful not to affect long hairs in your perfect line. In those cases, get out the mini scissors and trim, but don't pluck. If you grow outside of a great line, then feel free to tweeze. Frida Kahlo we are not! Use one shade lighter than your hair to draw on individual hairs or fill in the whole field. You may want to do a combination of individual lines with a brush of powder to create the best texture. Here is a general guideline:

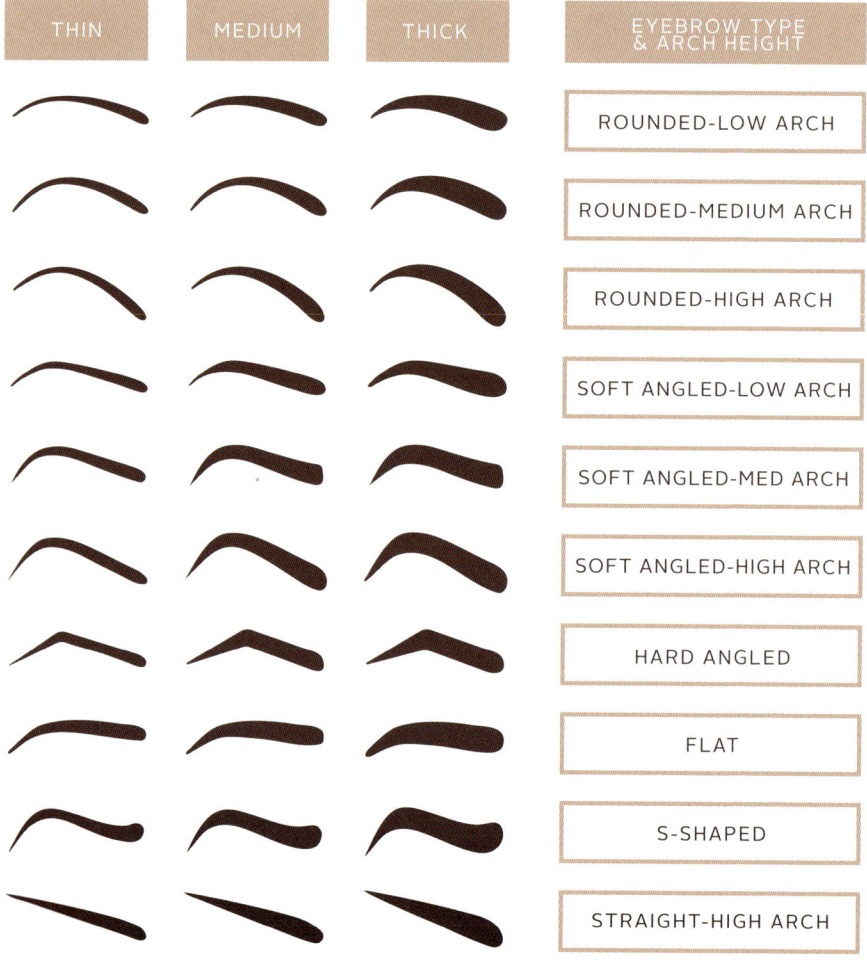

THIN	MEDIUM	THICK	EYEBROW TYPE & ARCH HEIGHT
			ROUNDED-LOW ARCH
			ROUNDED-MEDIUM ARCH
			ROUNDED-HIGH ARCH
			SOFT ANGLED-LOW ARCH
			SOFT ANGLED-MED ARCH
			SOFT ANGLED-HIGH ARCH
			HARD ANGLED
			FLAT
			S-SHAPED
			STRAIGHT-HIGH ARCH

Lip Shapes

The nineties were a love affair with lip liner. Cue the sad, sad crybaby music for the people who had lip liners tattooed, thinking that trend was here to stay. You can modify the shape of your lips with how you apply your lip dressing—whether that's Savvy gloss or lipstick. Just remember that drawing on clown lips (like the wax novelty ones we had as kids), will only bring laughs. And that's okay, if you're truly looking for them!

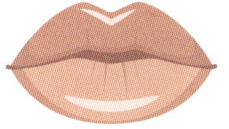

FULL LIPS

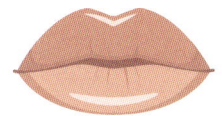

HEAVY UPPER LIPS

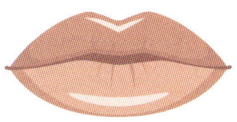

WIDE LIPS

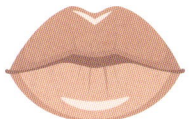

ROUND LIPS

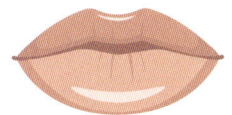

HEAVY LOWER LIPS

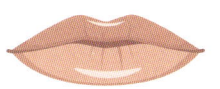

THIN LIPS

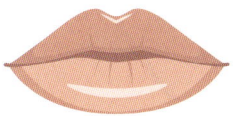

BOW-SHAPED LIPS

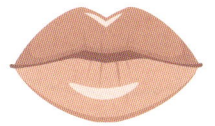

HEART-SHAPED LIPS

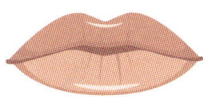

DOWN-TURNED LIPS

Your Basic 5-Minute Face

The pages that directly follow are for you to explore what products and colors you'd like to use on your own face. Fill in your own face facts. Then feel free to experiment and capture your favorite combinations.

Face Shape _____
Eye Shape _____
Lip Shape _____
Brow Shape _____
Care _____
Cleanser _____
Serum _____
Special Care_____

Eye Cream _____
Face Cream _____
Eye Shape _____
Correction _____
Treatment _____
Concealer _____
Foundation 1 _____
Foundation 2 _____

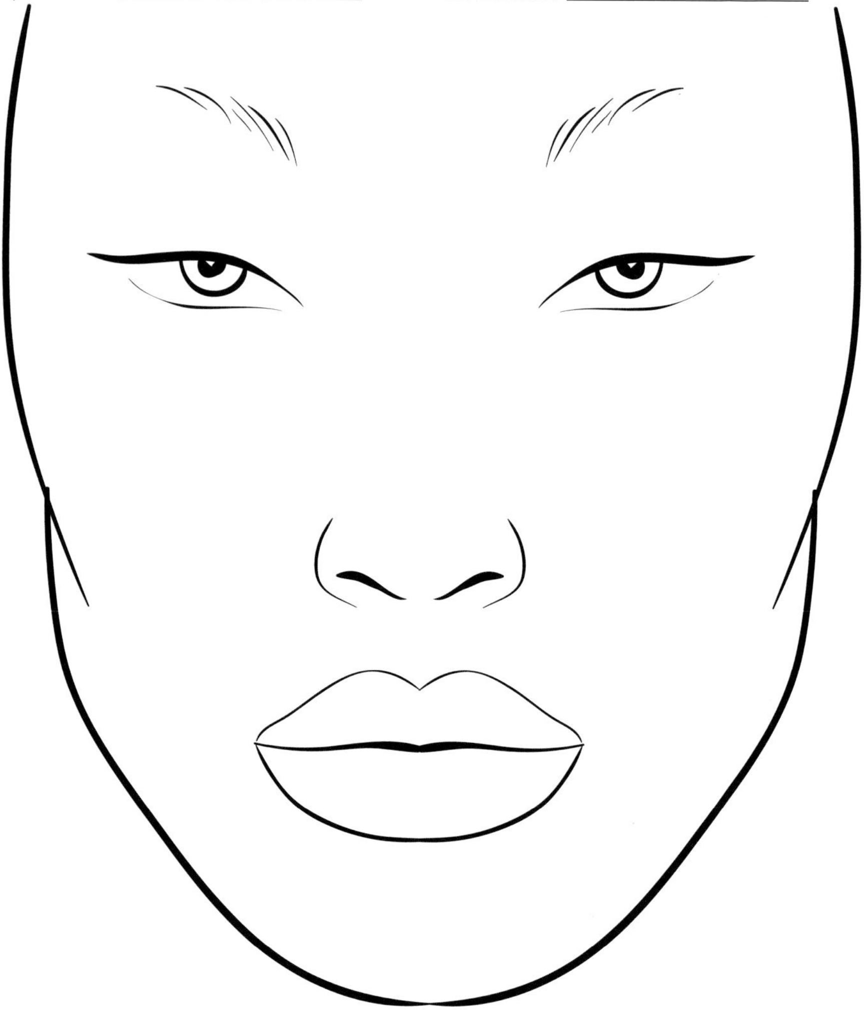

Brushes _____
Blush _____
Bronzer _____
Highlighter _____
Shading _____
Contouring _____
Lips _____
Color _____

Eyes _____
Liner _____
Lid _____
Crease _____
Lower Lid _____
Brushes _____
Mascara _____
Finishing _____

Face Shape _____
Eye Shape _____
Lip Shape _____
Brow Shape _____
Care _____
Cleanser _____
Serum _____
Special Care _____

Eye Cream _____
Face Cream _____
Eye Shape _____
Correction _____
Treatment _____
Concealer _____
Foundation 1 _____
Foundation 2 _____

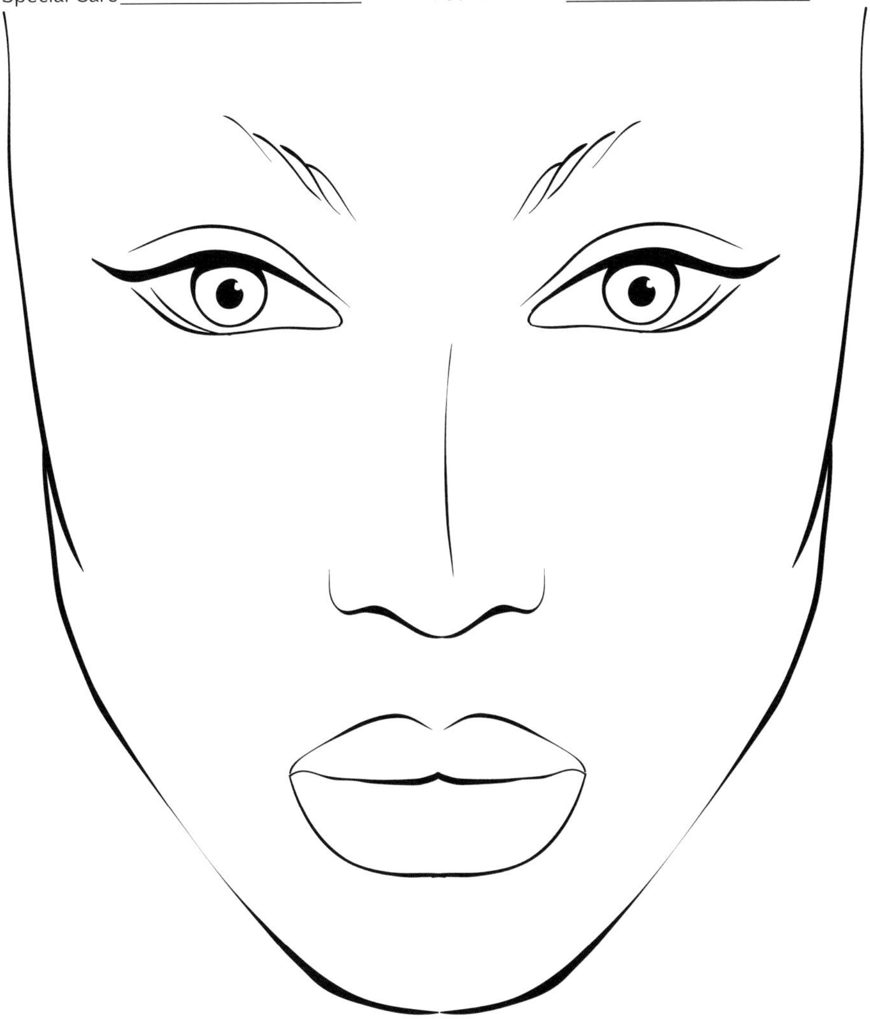

Brushes _____
Blush _____
Bronzer _____
Highlighter _____
Shading _____
Contouring _____
Lips _____
Color _____

Eyes _____
Liner _____
Lid _____
Crease _____
Lower Lid _____
Brushes _____
Mascara _____
Finishing _____

Face Shape _____   Eye Cream _____
Eye Shape _____   Face Cream _____
Lip Shape _____   Eye Shape _____
Brow Shape _____   Correction _____
Care _____   Treatment _____
Cleanser _____   Concealer _____
Serum _____   Foundation 1 _____
Special Care _____   Foundation 2 _____

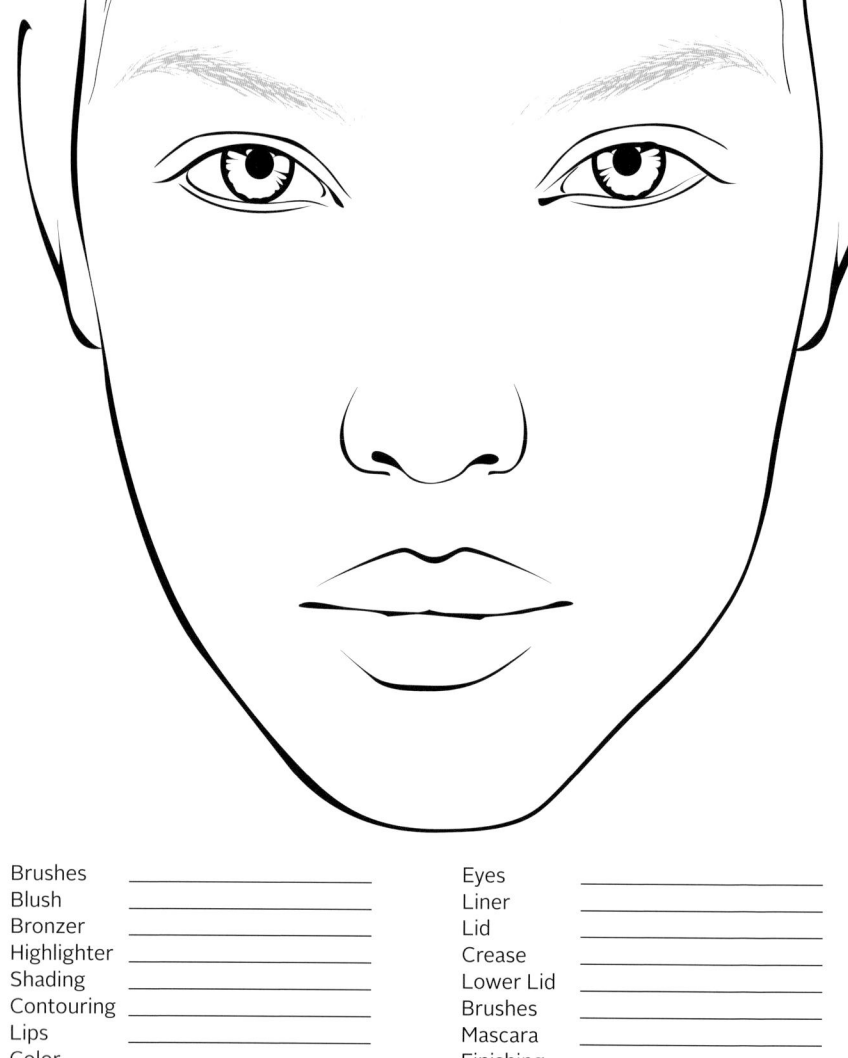

Brushes _____   Eyes _____
Blush _____   Liner _____
Bronzer _____   Lid _____
Highlighter _____   Crease _____
Shading _____   Lower Lid _____
Contouring _____   Brushes _____
Lips _____   Mascara _____
Color _____   Finishing _____

Face Shape _____
Eye Shape _____
Lip Shape _____
Brow Shape _____
Care _____
Cleanser _____
Serum _____
Special Care _____

Eye Cream _____
Face Cream _____
Eye Shape _____
Correction _____
Treatment _____
Concealer _____
Foundation 1 _____
Foundation 2 _____

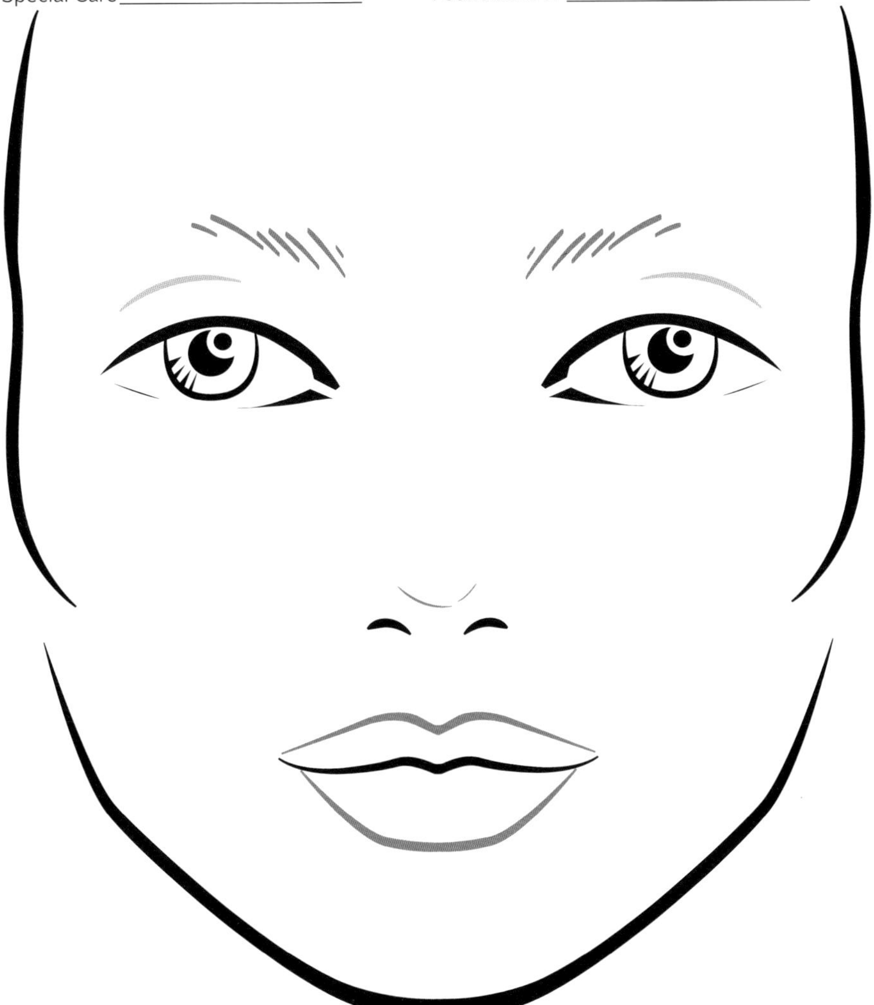

Brushes _____
Blush _____
Bronzer _____
Highlighter _____
Shading _____
Contouring _____
Lips _____
Color _____

Eyes _____
Liner _____
Lid _____
Crease _____
Lower Lid _____
Brushes _____
Mascara _____
Finishing _____

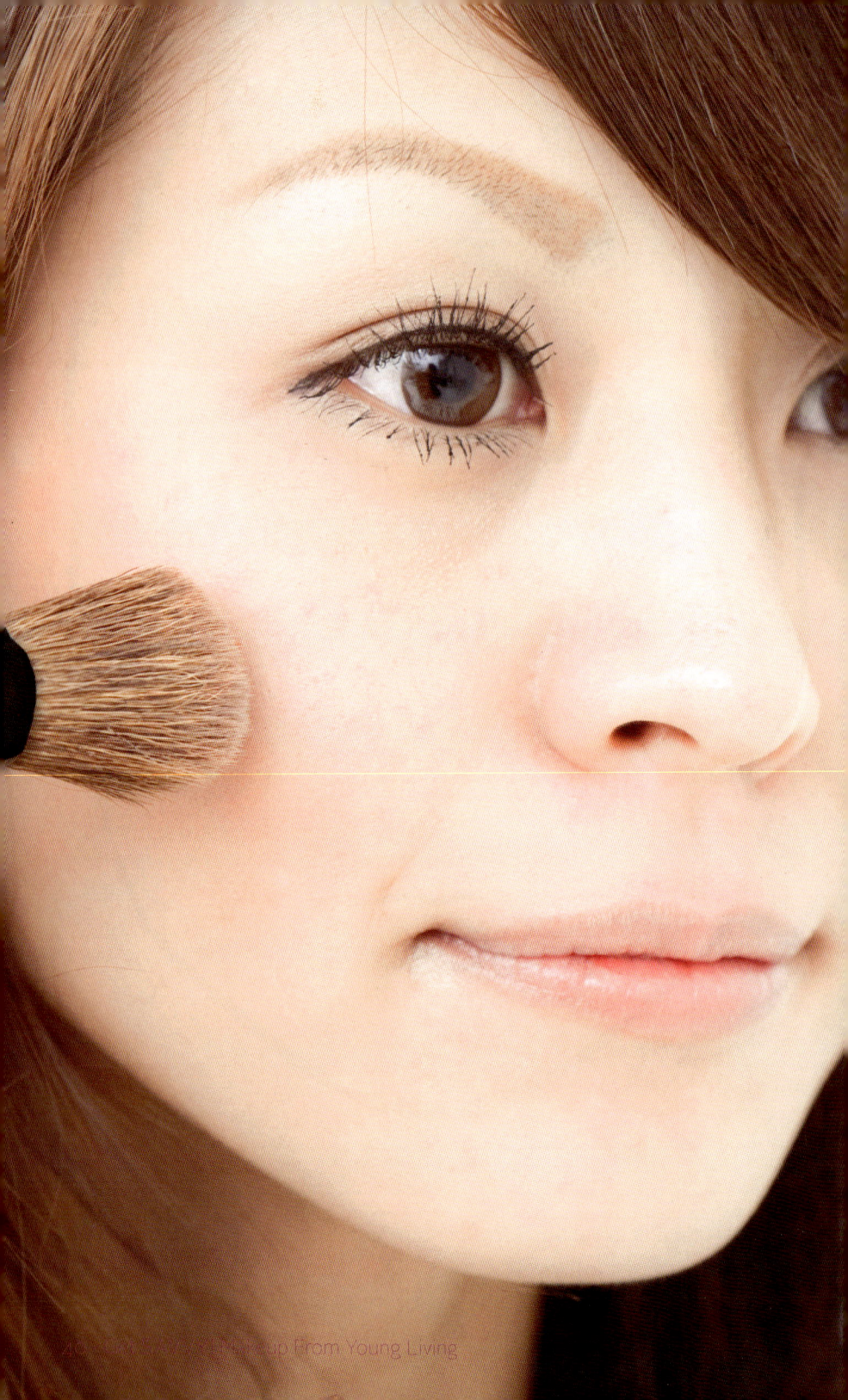

Foundation

The goal with foundation is to perfectly match your skin tone. Since Savvy Minerals is *Buildable, Blendable, & Forgiving*, you have a little wiggle room. Go from *Sheer to Full Coverage* with a few simple steps...

FIND YOUR SHADE

Savvy Mineral Foundation comes in 3 different tones—Warm, Cool, and Dark. Each tone has multiple shades. Higher numbers are darker shades. So, the lightest colors will be labeled "1" such as Cool number 1, Warm number 1, and Dark number 1.

START WITH YOUR UNDERTONE

• A Warm undertone equates to gold, peach, or yellow.

• A Cool undertone is more red or pink.

• Look to your forearm as a cue. Do the veins look green or blue? If blue, you're cool. If green, you're warm.

• Take a tip from your natural eye and hair color. If you have blue, green, or gray eyes and have brown, blond, or black hair with violet, blue, silver or ash undertones, you're Cool. If you have amber, brown, or hazel eyes with red, brown, strawberry blond, or black hair, you're Warm.

• Match to the skin on the face above the jawline.

• If you feel you're in-between undertones, you might try blending the two in each tone that are closest to you. That may get you spot-on.

• When you tan, does it look golden or brown? Or, do you feel more ruddy, like you turn pink and then burn? The former is Warm and the latter is Cool.

Hint: *Most people who look fabulous in platinum or silver jewelry have cool undertones. Most people who look their best in gold jewelry have warm undertones.*

GO FOR TWO

Because our skin has more than one color to it, I always recommend using two shades. With the natural seasons, and even with sunblock, our skin changes shades throughout the year. This way, you always have a built-in plan for those changes as well as the ability to mix. Now, due to the inherent mixability, you can always use your bronzer and blush to tint your powder foundation color one way or the other. If it disappears on your face, you know you've found the right color.

PUTTING IT ON

The Savvy line is meant to go on with a brush strategy, but if you're a sponge user, try your own method first. You can always experiment or branch out. People who "bake" their powder on and have great results (without crinkling or looking like a raisin) should use Savvy the same way.

APPLY FOUNDATION

1. Spray 2–3 pumps of Savvy Mineral Misting Spray onto your makeup brush and gently wipe off any excess moisture, using the back of your hand.

2. Tap foundation minerals into the foundation cap.

3. Pick up mineral makeup, using the brush with a gentle swirling motion.

4. Apply the foundation to your desired facial areas in gentle circular motions. Apply additional layers to build coverage. Re-apply in thin layers throughout the day as needed.

PRIMING

Nothing gives you more even coverage than gently applying a priming layer of ART Renewal Serum and ART Light Moisturizer over your whole face.

LIQUID/CREME FOUNDATION

Many creme foundations are preferred for skin of a certain age. If you're a die-hard for liquids, have no fear. You can still take 1-2 pumps ART Light/Intensive Moisturizer and mix the foundation powder to your desired consistency. The beauty is that you have some freedom to adjust color this way as well.

Feel free to use Wolfberry Eye Cream, ART Renewal Serum, Mineral Sunscreen, Sheerlumé, Sandalwood Moisture Cream, or ART Creme Masque the same way. It's your skin, your makeup, your beautiful face. Do with it as you will to make it feel its best.

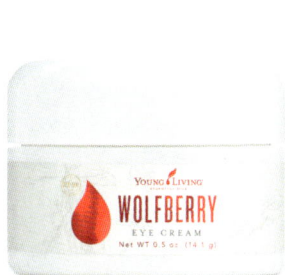

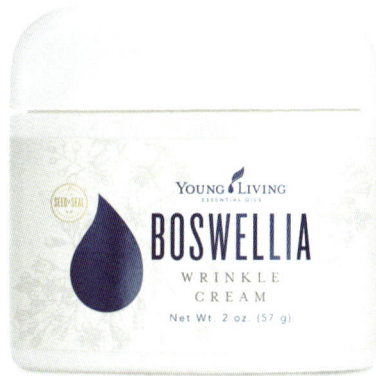

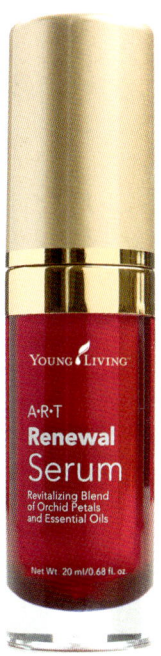

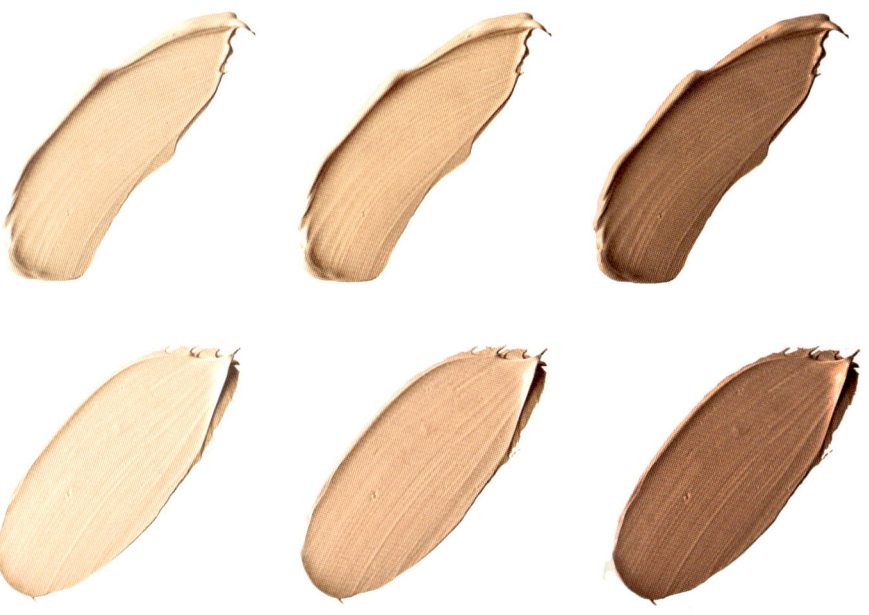

Concealing

The challenge for many people with Savvy Minerals is figuring out how to conceal. As of this printing, there is no dedicated concealer in the line. For many of us with dark circes under our eyes, broken capillaries, pimples, or blemishes, this can be troublesome.

There are some ways to get the coverage you want with the powder foundation, however. For under eyes, the popular "baking" method can work. Start with Rose Ointment or Wolfberry Eye Cream under the eyes. Using your brush or damp sponge, add a layer of foundation powder under the eye over the top of the emoillient you decide to use. Over-apply and allow the excess to stay on and "bake" through for 10 minutes. Once time is up, brush away excess, and blend with a new layer all over the face.

You can also create your own using the Young Living cream of your choice mixed with your powder foundation. Use a 1:1 ratio to start. Then add more or less powder to your mix, depending on your preferred consistency. Dab on the way you ordinarily would with a cream concealer. Blend well. Apply foundation powder over the top for increased covereage.

Stippling

You don't *always* need to add *full* foundation, all over your face, all of the time. If you want to use fewer layers of Savvy Minerals powder foundation, you can always use your concealer brush to dab smaller, more concentrated bits of foundation to your trouble area. Tap it on the area with your brush. Then tap it out with your finger. That will help it blend with the surrounding skin. Repeat the process until the blemish disappears. Follow it up with an all-over layer of powder foundation.

Lighting

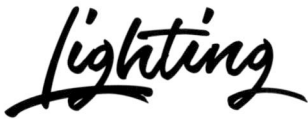

Remember: lighting is EVERYTHING. Colors will switch in different lighting. To apply your best, always do so in the harshest light in which you think you'll appear. That way, your match is sound, and you don't stumble into the unexpected or into a "YIKES" moment!

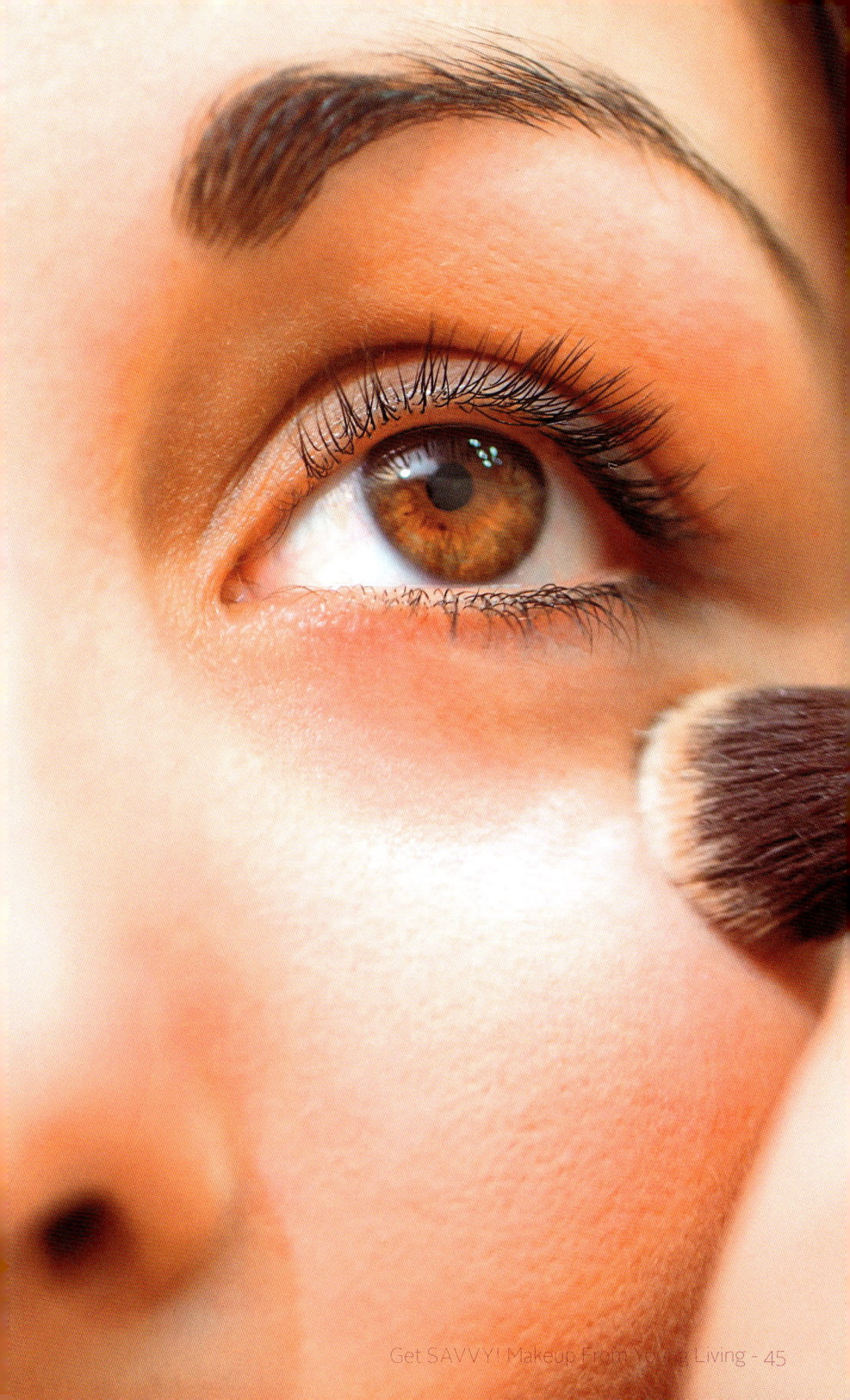

Contouring

Contouring doesn't have to be scary. Just don't scare anyone with your unblended contouring. (Great look for Halloween, not for every day, LOL!)

1. THROW SOME SHADE
Start by assessing your shadows. Using the guideline chart, work with what nature gave you. If you want your cheekbones to bump up a little, try to determine where the natural shadows would actually fall. This is usually the area directly underneath your cheekbones, extending to the top of the jawline. If you want to minimize your nose bridge, apply shading to the sides of the nose. Finish out shading with the top of your hairline. Apply a line of contouring makeup (either bronzer or darker shade of Savvy powder foundation) in each of these places.

2. LET IN THE LIGHT
Then it's time to highlight. Since you've created the illusion of shadows, you'll want to shine the light on your face strategically. Use a highlighting color (at least 1 shade lighter than your main foundation), brush your lighter powder across the tops of your cheekbones and to the center of your face to bring those features forward.

3. BLEND AWAY
Finally, blend and go. Use a blending brush, smooth out the contour and highlighter lines and ensure a natural, polished look.

There. It's that simple!

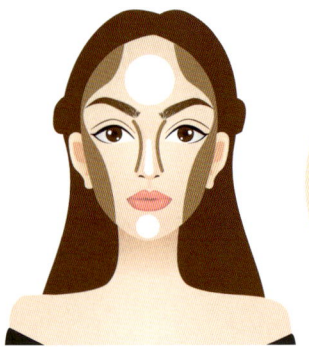

OVAL

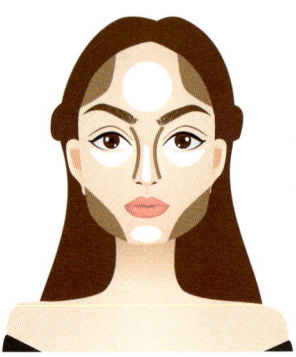

SQUARE

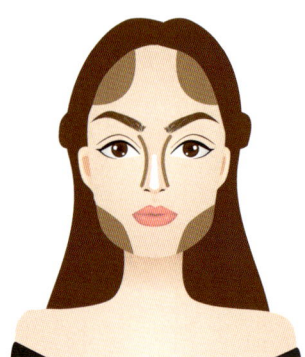

RECTANGLE

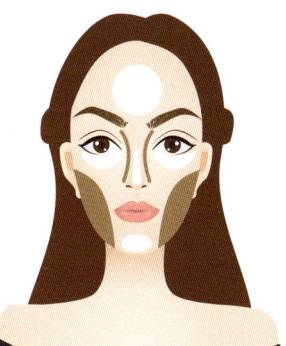

OBLONG

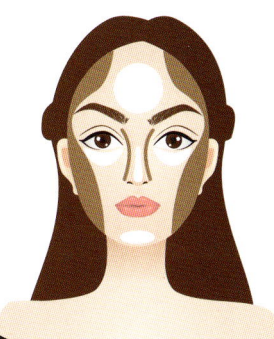

ROUND

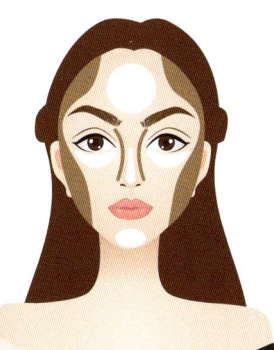

HEART

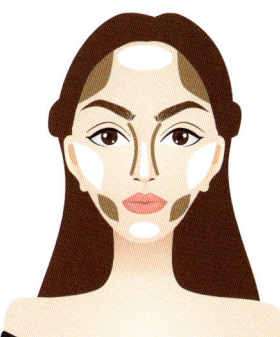

DIAMOND

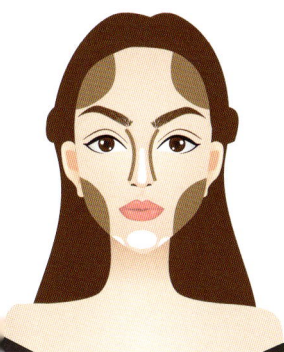

TRIANGLE

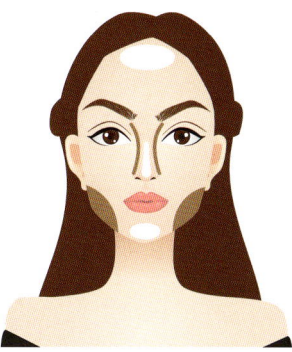

HEPTAGON

Eye Lining

How you line your eyes is as important as *whether or not you decide* to line them at all. You can absolutely transform your look by transforming your lining strategy. Just remember, there's a time and place for Cleopatra.

Almond: Go for Basic, Simple, Dropped Flick, Egyptian, Open Wings, Soft Smoke, Feline, Arabic, Slept-in Smudge, Pin-Up, Double Flick, Luxe, Double Up, Classic Bar, Bold, Double Mod, Drama, or Panda Smudge.

Downturned: Go for Egyptian, Feline, Pin-Up, Double Flick, Classic Bar, Bold, or Double Mod.

Upturned: Go for Basic, Simple, Dropped Flick, Egyptian, Open Wings, Soft Smoke, Feline, Arabic, Slept-in Smudge, Pin-Up, Double Flick, Luxe, Double Up, Classic Bar, Bold, Double Mod, Drama, or Panda Smudge.

Close-Set: Go for Egyptian, Open Wings, Soft Smoke, Feline, Arabic, Slept-in Smudge, Pin-Up, Double Flick, Luxe, Double Up, Bold, Double Mod, Drama, or Panda Smudge.

Wide-Set: Go for Basic, Simple, Dropped Flick, Egyptian, Luxe, Double Mod, Drama, or Panda Smudge.

Round: Go for Basic, Simple, Dropped Flick, Open Wings, Soft Smoke, Feline, Arabic, Slept-in Smudge, Pin-Up, Double Flick, Double Up, Classic Bar, Bold, Double Mod, or Drama.

Protruding: Go for Egyptian, Open Wings, Soft Smoke, Feline, Arabic, Slept-In Smudge, Double up, Pin-Up, Double Flick, Bold, or Double Mod.

Hooded: Go for Basic, Egyptian, Open Wings, Soft Smoke, Feline, Arabic, Slept-in Smudge, Pin-Up, Double Flick, Luxe, Double Up, Double Mod, Drama, or Panda Smudge.

Monolid: Go for Basic, Simple, Dropped Flick, Egyptian, Open Wings, Soft Smoke, Feline, Arabic, Slept-in Smudge, Pin-Up, Double Flick, Luxe, Double Up, Classic Bar, Bold, Double Mod, Drama, or Panda Smudge.

All Types of Liner Reference

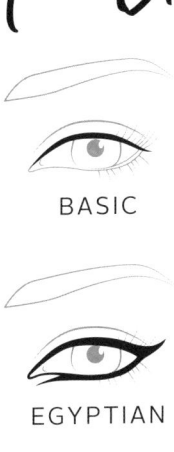

BASIC

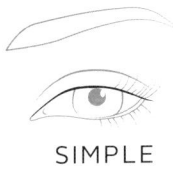

SIMPLE

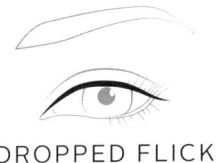

DROPPED FLICK

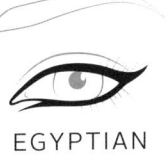

EGYPTIAN

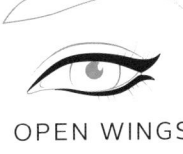

OPEN WINGS

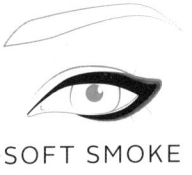

SOFT SMOKE

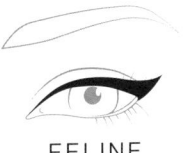

FELINE

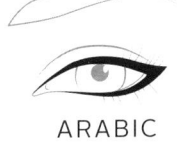

ARABIC

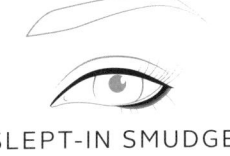

SLEPT-IN SMUDGE

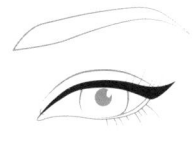

PIN-UP

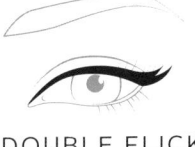

DOUBLE FLICK

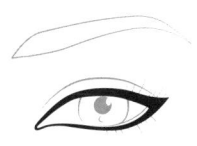

LUXE

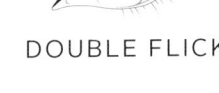

DOUBLE UP

CLASSIC BAR

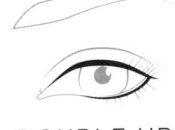

DOUBLE UP

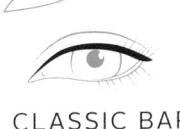

CLASSIC BAR

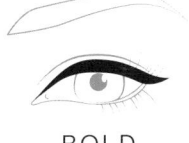

BOLD

DOUBLE MOD

DRAMA

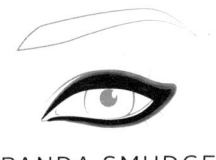

PANDA SMUDGE

Eyelashes

MASCARA

Mascara is one of those things we all love. In fact, it's kind of the *deserted island* answer if you could only have one thing (aside from sunscreen, perhaps). Survivor scenarios aside, we really tend to love our mascara, and we consume it quickly (as we should for hygenic reasons). It's also one of the most important things that should be absolutely toxin-free, because we we put it so close to our eye ducts. That's a huge concern for absorption into the body!

Mascara should be conditioning to the eyelash itself. In other words, it should really boost the natural health of your lashes and ducts. If it doesn't do that, you're missing an opportunity. The only trouble is, there's only one brand that can really make claim to that benefit. So, we're a little stuck with one option.

Since we're all putting that demand on our Savvy Minerals, at the time of this printing, Savvy mascara is sold out. This is bound to happen with healthy things that work—and people happen to LOVE! And, it will likely happen from time to time, since supply for Young Living product is so organic and standards-driven.

USING SAVVY MASCARA

Using Savvy Minerals mascara is pretty straightforward. Start with a really clean brush. No one wants a clumpy wad. If you apply with one, you'll only have a mess. If you're concerned about wasting product, try cleaning the brush off into the top of the mascara pot. Then, wipe the brush off on a clean tissue or damp cloth.

Next, apply at an angle. Start at the base. Wiggle back and forth as you brush outward to maximize your volume. By doing it at an angle , you can be sure to hit every lash. With the shape of your eyes, you'll probably have to do two angles with each coating, particularly for the harder-to-reach areas at the edge.

Always be sure to wiggle across the roots. That's where you're going to get the most bang for your buck.

I recommend starting with your bottom lashes, if you happen to do your bottom lashes. If your eye shape looks odd, do only the top. Sometimes the flaking and the shadowing on the lower eyelid aren't worth the benefit. Give it a rest between coats. Allowing the coat to dry will really boost your results with each pass. Some artists would recommend around five coats. If you're going more than three, you'll want to use an eyelash comb.

For even thicker lashes, try applying a layer of Veil Powder (Diamont Dust) to your lashes between coats.

CURLING

It's not just an interesting Olympic sport. As long as you are gentle and use a quality tool, I recommend curling your lashes. Do it between coats. Start from the roots, and be careful. You usually don't need to do it every day. A couple of times a week may work if your lashes are in good condition. If your lashes aren't, try blinking a sterile drop of coconut oil on them each night before bed. Do this with a cotton swab or clean, specifically-devoted brush.

MAKING YOUR OWN

When supply can't meet demand, you can actually make a version of your own mascara using to tide you over in a couple of different ways.

FLAT BRUSH / BLINK ON

Taking a clean, flat glass lip balm holder, add 1/8 teaspoon of Jetsetter or Multitasker. Next, dip a clean flat brush in distilled water and mix it around the glass lip balm holder, carefully mising the pigment. Now, act as though you are going to line the wet line of your eye, but as you touch the base of the lash line, simply blink the color onto your lashes. Repeat the process until you have enough color. Use a cotton swab to fix any splashover or blinked-off droplets.

TRADITIONAL RECIPE/METHOD

Using one of your old Savvy mascara bottles (or a new, generic, empty one, if you like), clean the inside and out with very hot water. Use a drop or two of Thieves to really clean the brush and inside of the bottle. Then, using a small funnel and 1/8 teaspoon measurer, pour 1/8 teaspoon of Jetsetter or Multitasker into the funnel (you can get these tiny ones from Life Science Publishing: discoverlsp.com) and into the bottle.

Next, add 1 drop of Lavender and 10 drops of fractionated coconut oil. Finally, add three 1/8 teaspoons of distilled water. Follow with 1/8 teaspoon of fine-grade kaolin clay powder or Veil Powder (Diamond Dust). Put the brush top on to seal, and shake well. Mix thoroughly with the brush to stir around. Shake/mix each time you use.

Basic Acne Read*

As you suffer the occasional breakout, most dermatologists will use this skin diagram (or one similar) as a guideline for ways you can help minimize the issue. While most blemishes are hormone and stress-related, there are some behavior changes that at least support clearer skin. While the answer for conventional doctors is a pharmaceutical, take a look at your own natural bevy of solutions and consider your options.

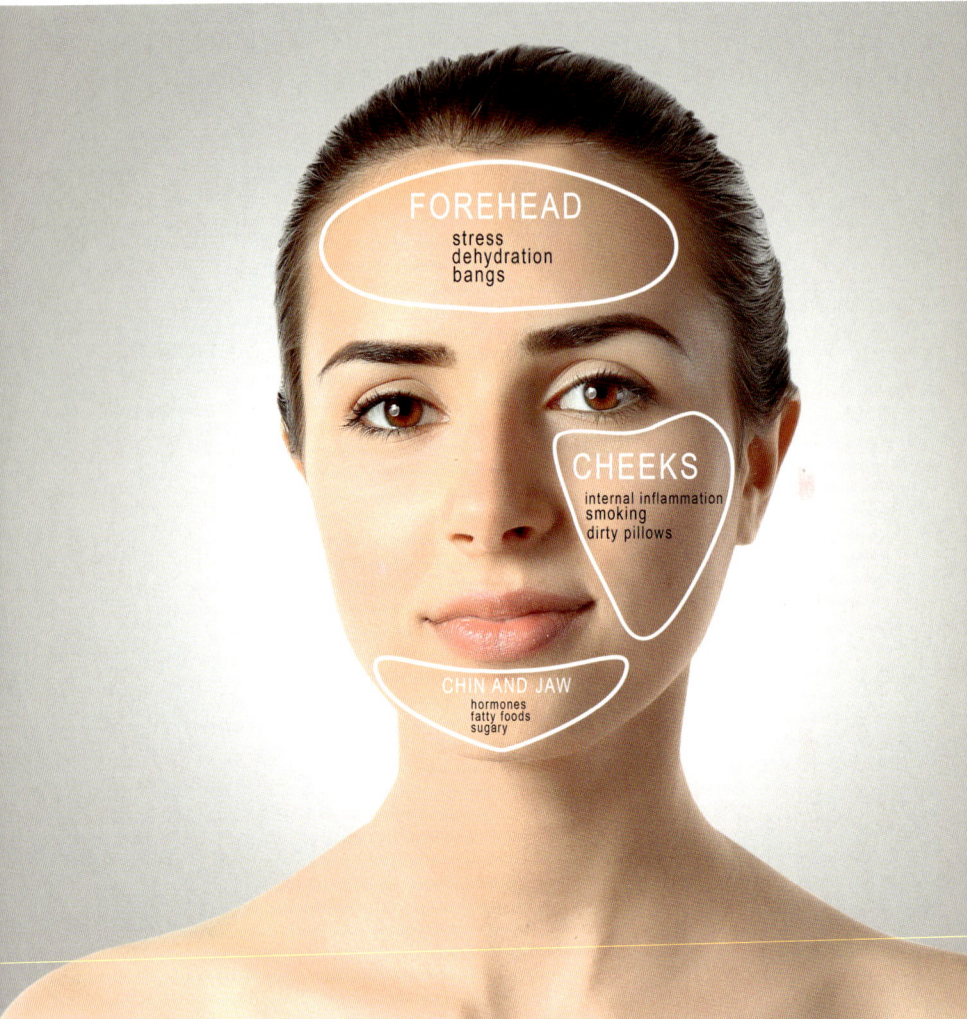

FOREHEAD
stress
dehydration
bangs

CHEEKS
internal inflammation
smoking
dirty pillows

CHIN AND JAW
hormones
fatty foods
sugary

*Not intended to diagnose, treat, cure, or prevent any disease.

Your Skin is Talking*...

ARE YOU LISTENING?

Beyond just acne, our makeup-less face can say a lot about our general health. Just like with Vita Flex for the feet, there are zones of the face in Traditional Chinese Medicine that correspond with the systems of the body. Part of being Savvy about your makeup and skincare is learning to listen to your body's cues and adjust accordingly. Look to your oils for support...

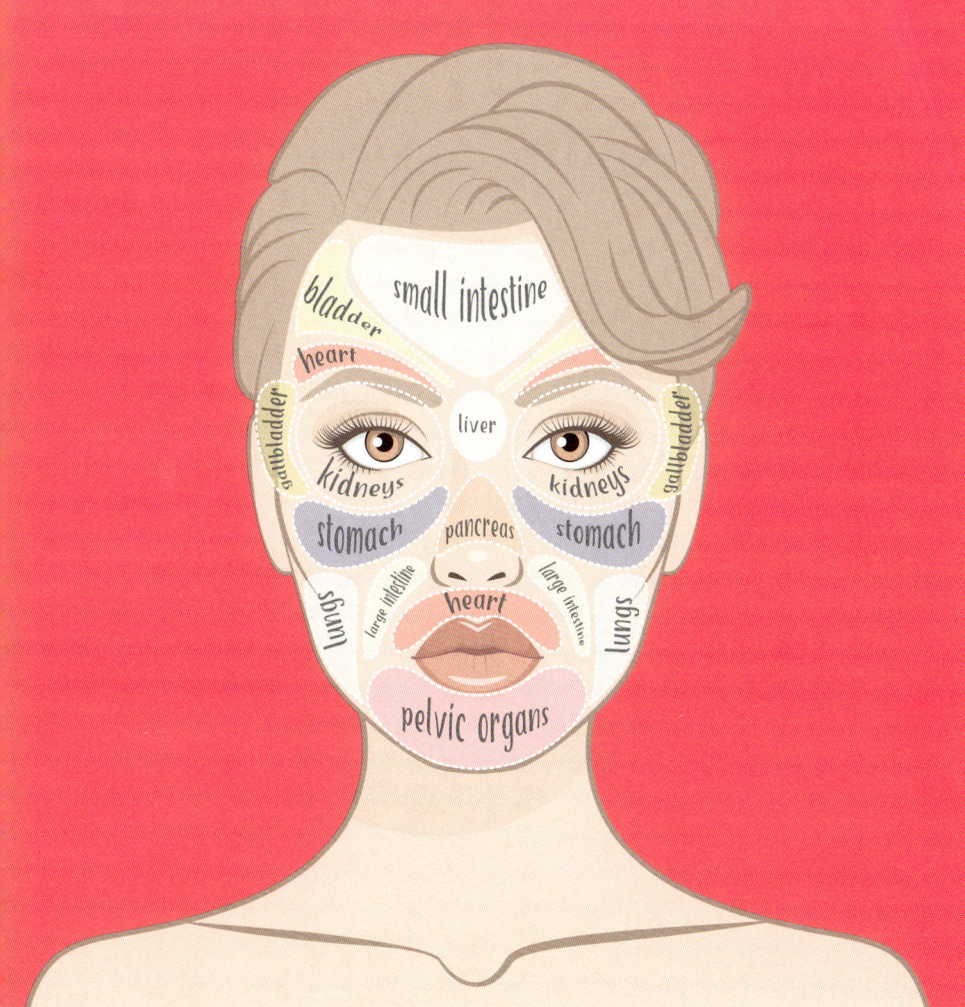

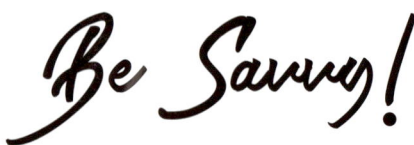

THE ARGUMENT FOR SAVVY

Okay, I'll say it. The only makeup you should buy is the kind that actually supports your skin's (and body's) overall health. Even more, you should only buy Otherwise, you're doing harm, right? The only makeup on the market that's truly toxin-free is Savvy Minerals. Therefore, the only makeup you should ever buy is...

See what I did there? I used that same argument your parents used to use when they expected you to come home with perfect grades. "Honey, we only want you to do your best. But, we know that your best is perfect..."
You're left to fill in the gap.

But seriously, there isn't anything on the market with as much transparency as Savvy Minerals. I've tried a zillion products, and though they work wonderfully, there's always a fatal flaw when it comes to a potentially toxic additive.

Don't take my word for it. Visit the Environmental Working Group's (EWG) *Skin Deep Database* or try the *Think Dirty* App to get a better sense of all the problematic ingredients in your current makeup.

All makeup boils down to being a pigment mixed with a vehicle. By that, I mean, color mixed with something that can go onto the skin and blend. The beauty of Savvy Minerals is that you can not only use it the way the label says, but you have a lot of off-label ways of DIY (doing it yourself).

For example, perhaps you are more familiar with a cream foundation or water-based gel foundation? Great news! The pigments in Savvy Minerals will blend with other Young Living products (or even your favorite conventional products). The more you know, the more you self-educate, the more you experiment, the greater your possibilities. The sky is the limit. Truly.

The more savvy you get (or, the more Savvy you acquire), the cleaner and more natural your skin routine will be. The more product you acquire, the more creative you can be as you experiment on yourself and/or share the line with other people.

MARKET COMPARISON

So, when you think about the cost of Savvy Minerals and the value you enjoy from having a toxin-free brand, what does that look like? How much is "clean" makeup worth to you, personally?

Regardless of where you buy your makeup, a basic set for your daily face will likely include:

Young Living Savvy Minerals		Comparable Department Store		Average Young Living Premium Starter Kit	
Foundation	$44.00	Foundation	$35.00	(1) Foundation	$44.00
Blush	$27.75	Blush	$34.00	(1) Blush	$27.75
Eyeliner	$15.75	Eyeliner	$19.00	(3) Eyeshadows	$45.75
Eyeshadow	$15.25	Eyeshadow	$15.00	(1) Lip Gloss	$27.50
Lip Gloss	$27.50	Lip Gloss	$18.00	(1) Misting Spray	$15.00
Lipstick	$22.75	Lipstick	$20.00	(1) Foundation Brush	$34.00
	Total=$150 .00		Total=$141.00	+(1) 5 ml Lavender	$12.00

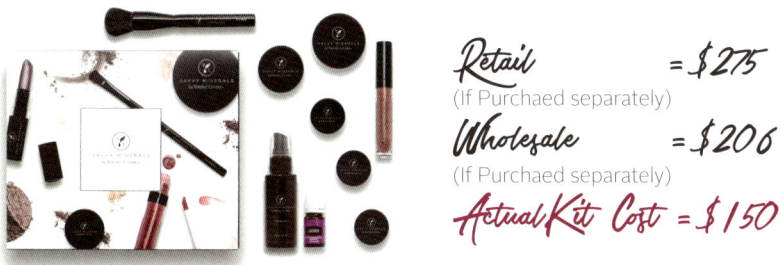

Retail = $275
(If Purchaed separately)

Wholesale = $206
(If Purchaed separately)

Actual Kit Cost = $150

As you can see, the cost is pretty comparable to higher-end department store brands. The difference with Young Living is that you have a Seed to Seal guarantee as well as toxin-free formulation. Other brands won't give you points in the form of Essential Rewards, nor will you earn PV when you shop the makeup counter. Those can add up to as much as 25% once you've worked your way up the longevity ladder. And, what company will give that back to you in rewards you can spend? Hint: you won't find that deal at the fancy schmancy makeup counter.

Most of us will choose our health and long-term quality of life over questionable ingredients. Yes, you can be beautiful for less, but how long will that last?

PLAN & SAVE

Whether you're changing up your Essential Rewards (ER) order, or you're just thinking about getting a Premium Starter Kit (PSK), with a little planning, you can get a wonderful deal on great makeup that comes with little-to-no guilt or worry.

The great news is that Young Living has assembled exactly what you need in 4 different Premium Starter Kits (as of the time of this printing). You owe it to yourself to try one. Try one with a friend and do two different sets. Then, using some of the small salve and lip balm jars from Life Science Publishing, split the colors between you and double your color options!

The point is to BE SAVVY!

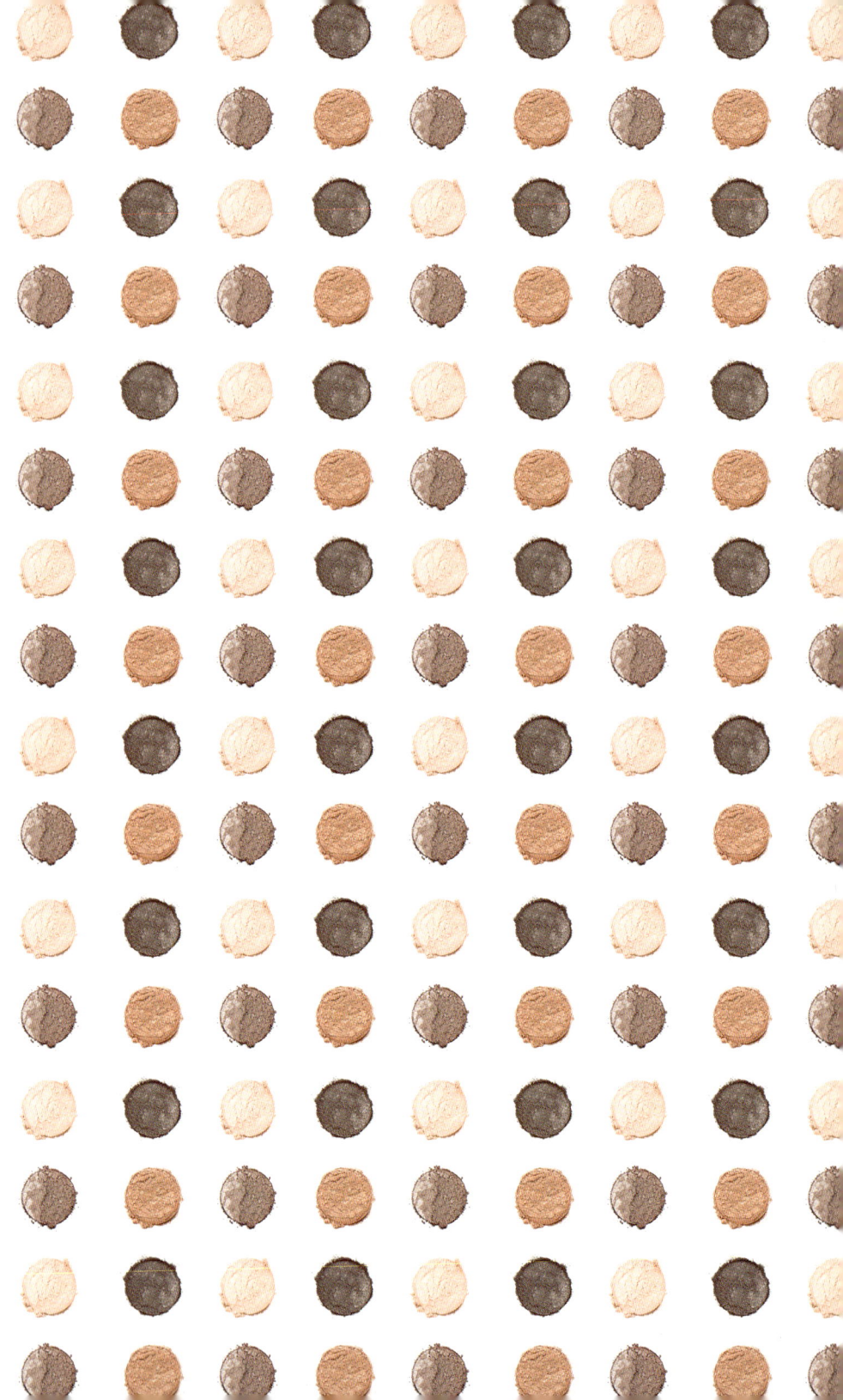